C000059249

Parents an

Parents and Bereavement

A personal and professional exploration of grief

Christine Young and
Tracy Dowling

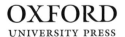

OXFORD
UNIVERSITY PRESS

Great Clarendon Street, Oxford, OX2 6DP,
United Kingdom

Oxford University Press is a department of the University of Oxford.
It furthers the University's objective of excellence in research, scholarship,
and education by publishing worldwide. Oxford is a registered trade mark of
Oxford University Press in the UK and in certain other countries

First Edition published in 2012

Impression: 1

British Library Cataloguing in Publication Data

Data available

Library of Congress Cataloging in Publication Data

Data available

ISBN 978–0–19–965264–8

Printed and bound by
CPI Group (UK) Ltd, Croydon, CR0 4YY

Dedication

For Tom and Charlie

Foreword

Dr Su Laurent

Barnet and Chase Farm Hospitals Trust and
Consultant Paediatrician and Trustee of the Child
Bereavement Charity

I first met Tracy when Tom was four years old. Tom was very unwell and I didn't know then but it was the start of a very long relationship, initially as doctor and parent and now as friends and mutual supporters. As a paediatrician, I have learnt a huge amount from Tracy: the strength she found to support Tom through his devastating, debilitating illness, her ability to get the best out of health professionals and enable us to work together, and her skill in asking the right questions in order to understand what was happening to her son. I am delighted that she now uses her wisdom and strength both to support bereaved parents and to train junior doctors in how to support grieving families. In this book Tracy describes the painful and difficult times she and her family went through and highlights the things she found helpful in order to help others going through bereavement. She talks about things others did, often only small gestures, which really helped, and contrasts these with insensitive things people may say, often without realizing it. She describes how she coped with facing people in everyday situations. The way in which Tracy describes preparing for Tom's death with such dignity and courage is a lesson for all professionals in how to work together in partnership with families.

In each chapter, after Tracy describes an aspect of her journey since Tom's death, Christine uses her experience as a counsellor to explain the process of grief in order to make sense of how she was feeling. She refers to wide ranging research in the area of bereavement and writes about it in a very readable way. She discusses the range of emotions parents may feel and how they may rapidly move from one to another. She uses examples from the parents she has supported to describe their journeys and to demonstrate the normal aspects of grief such as guilt, the intense physical pain, and the feeling many parents have of going mad. Each chapter ends with a list of bullet points to help you remember the key ideas.

What shines out of this book for me is hope. Both Tracy and Christine demonstrate how, eventually, families learn to live with their loss rather than be overwhelmed by it. They show how it is possible to continue living through their grief. The combination of Tracy's first-hand experience and Christine's training, skill, and knowledge in supporting families through the death of a child makes this book a 'must read' for both parents and professionals.

Acknowledgements

We would like to thank Helen and Douglas House for encouraging us with this project and for their support throughout. The insights and suggestions of friends and colleagues working there were immensely helpful. Our greatest thanks, however, go to the many families from whom we have learned so much through individual conversations and in the groups and workshops. Special thanks are owed to those parents who allowed us to write about their experiences and to those who read the text and offered very constructive feedback. We could not have written this without you. Neither could it have been completed without patience and understanding on the home front and for this Christine thanks Alex, Jamie and Ross.

Helen and Douglas House

Helen and Douglas House has the time and expertise to care for children and young adults with life-shortening conditions and support their families. The two hospice houses offer specialist symptom and pain management, medically-supported short breaks and end-of-life care, as well as counselling and practical support for the whole family.

Our aim is to help every young person—aged from birth to 35—who visits us from Oxfordshire and surrounding counties, live life to the full...even when that life is short.

W: www.helenanddouglas.org.uk T: 01865 794749
E: reception@helenanddouglas.org.uk
Registered charity number: 1085951

Contents

Introduction

Parent's Perspective

'You can go now, Sweetheart.'

When my son, Tom, died in April 2006 it was as though he needed my permission. I was lying in his bed beside him, listening to his breathing become shallower, stroking his skin, and breathing in the smell of his hair. Yet still he fought it.

He had been very unwell with a chest infection for nearly two weeks and he just kept defying his doctors and nurses. He was at home in his own bed, and I had sat with him almost constantly for the previous ten days. Over that period of time family and friends were given the opportunity to visit and perhaps say their goodbyes. Something within me allowed myself to unknowingly share what was such an emotional time. During his last few hours I was able to spend time alone with him, talking about things we had done and the people we had done it all with. I told him how proud I was of him and that I loved him more than I could ever find the words to tell him. I told him that it was OK for him to go now, that I would be OK; that his little brother, Charlie, who was nine years old, would be OK. Tom died a short while after, peacefully with my arms around him.

I had nearly lost Tom before. More than once in fact. He was nearly thirteen years old and was severely disabled as a result of a catastrophic brain injury when he was just four. Then, two days after being admitted into our local hospital with an E. coli infection, he was rushed into Great Ormond Street Hospital where he fell into a coma and spent twelve days in intensive care. His prognosis was very poor, and I was told that it was unlikely that he would survive the massive bleed he had sustained in his brain. But, it seemed, Tom was not having any of that. He wasn't ready to go. He survived, but his injury left him profoundly disabled, unable to eat or talk and with epilepsy. He remained in hospital for almost two years, during which time I was able to organize a life for him to come home to again.

Once home at last, I felt compelled to pack as much into what I knew would be a short life for Tom. I meticulously planned and provided for him. The last nine years of his life had been an uphill struggle to try to regain lost skills and to find a new way of family life.

As he got older, his disabilities and the extent of the damage to his body from the initial illness began to take their toll and after many hours of honest conversations with the medical team who provided us with care and support, I was able to think about how I would want Tom to die. Just writing that makes a monstrous feeling raise its head within me. How on earth could a mother want her child to die?

This is the thing: I didn't want Tom to die but I had to come to terms with the horrible reality that it was going to happen. The coping skills I had developed over those previous difficult years kicked in and it became obvious that there were certain things I was sure I didn't want to happen.

I didn't want Tom dying in A&E, on a trolley, having been rushed in from somewhere by ambulance. I didn't want Tom to die in intensive care, after he had been ventilated for some time, and then having to make the hideous decision that nothing more could be done for him. I had to accept that the quality of his life had to make up for its cruel lack of quantity.

After much discussion I decided that I wanted Tom to be at home. I feel eternally grateful to this day that I was allowed this privilege. I am grateful that nobody had to break the news of his death to me. I am grateful that we were as close then as the day he was born. I am grateful that I had the support to be able to remain as calm as I could be and to cherish those last days and hours.

In this book, I would like to share my experience of how it felt to lose that most precious of things – the child I brought into this world – and how I have survived the most painful of life's events.

I will talk about what I found useful in the first two years of my bereavement and also the flip side of what I found almost too much to bear. I will talk about how it felt to have lost every reason to get up each morning and how to survive the aftermath of such a loss. I will try and explain how I came to find a new identity when it felt like I had been stripped of my purpose in life.

This book is aimed at parents who have lost a child or who may be anticipating the loss of a life-limited child. It is not a book that will tell you how to get over the loss of a child; it is a book that will hopefully give you shared ideas on how to live with the loss of a child.

I am fully aware that grief is an extremely personal and individual experience, but having had the opportunity to share my experiences with other bereaved parents I have come to realize that there are many common threads. By including a chapter about how friends and family can support bereaved parents, we hope that this book will be useful to the wider family network.

I hope it will give you permission to feel the way it feels when you are grieving for your child. I often found I needed permission to enjoy myself or even laugh again. More often than not, it had to be given by myself. The most important decision I ever made was not to waste any energy in getting over the loss of my child; instead I gave myself permission to learn to live with the loss.

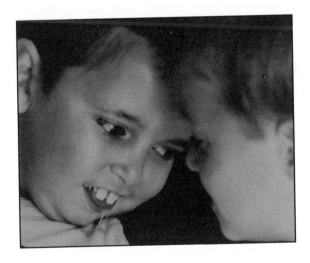

Professional Perspective

I met Tracy Dowling (Tom's mother) at Helen and Douglas House (a hospice for children and young adults in Oxford, UK), where I was then Head of Family Support and Bereavement. Several months after Tom's death she came to a workshop we were running for bereaved parents. She later joined a support group and also took up the offer of individual support, so for many months I had the privilege of visiting Tracy at home. In the course of these support sessions we discussed much of what we have now written about – the intense pain of loss and grief; how to support Charlie, Tom's younger brother; what Tracy needed from family and friends and what to do when she wasn't getting it; how to get through the significant days and events. Woven through all of these conversations were discussions about a future without Tom's physical presence and who this now meant Tracy was, or could be. As Tracy says, she gave herself permission to learn to live with the loss and that is what she has done and continues to do. She no longer needs my support, indeed it has not been needed for a while. We worked on other projects together – Tracy is one of the hospice's parent volunteers – and as I came up with the idea of writing this book, Tracy seemed the obvious parent to write it with. She had told me early on of coming across websites where ten or fifteen years on from their child's death parents were writing of their unchanged pain and anguish. She also told me that she had decided that she would not be one of those parents. And she has shown in what she shares in this book that her pain and her life have changed. In the past when I told people what my job was, I was often asked if it was depressing. My answer was always no, that while there are times when it is sad, this work is just the opposite of depressing. It is in fact life affirming. Tracy and all of the parents I have worked with have drawn on incredible inner strength to come to terms with the loss of their son or daughter and to cope with the changes wrought by the death. Supporting and witnessing that resilience brings hope, not despair.

We hope that by combining Tracy's own experience, creativity, and resilience with what I have learned from supporting other parents over the years we can help you make sense of what is happening to you and your family. There is no right way or wrong way to 'do' grief.

What we offer is neither a prescription nor a 'how to' manual, but a guide to get you through. We know that when you are grieving it is difficult to concentrate, so we have written the book in a style that is designed to allow you to dip in and out of it. Each chapter stands alone (with some cross-referencing) so that you can read it and understand it without having to read the whole book. We have included references and resources for those of you who want to find out more about a particular topic. Tracy begins each chapter with her personal experience and I follow on with an overview and suggestions for what might help. Your grief will be unique to you, but we hope that in some of the examples and experiences shared, there will be a glimmer of recognition that will encourage you to believe that you too will find your way through grief.

Chapter 1

What happens when we grieve?

Parent's Perspective

I 'celebrated' my birthday less than a month after Tom died, and I remember being taken out to dinner with a dozen or so of my close friends. I look back now at photographs of that evening and it is totally incomprehensible to me how I can be smiling and looking as though I am enjoying myself immensely. I can only assume that the numbness that set in during the early days of my grief lasted for some considerable time.

I recall having an unwelcome energy in those first few weeks that not only allowed me to plan Tom's funeral (meticulously, I might add, because I am a stickler for detail), but also to tackle some of the other tasks that I felt needed to be done sooner rather than later. I donated most of Tom's equipment to the rehabilitation unit where, nearly nine years earlier, he had spent eighteen months having therapy, telling myself that it was logical to do so while I still had a spacious, adapted vehicle to transport it. I cancelled the summer holiday we had booked and planned another one. It felt important that I had something to look forward to, even though I really couldn't face doing anything.

Looking back, it seems that I needed to undertake some practical jobs to make it feel as though my life was not completely useless. I needed to find ways of making sense of my loss, and by allowing other children to benefit from using Tom's specialist equipment it felt like something worthwhile. Having said that, I certainly wasn't ready to start redistributing all of Tom's things—only the things that were behind closed doors as it were. Tom's bedroom remains the same today; his clothes are still neatly folded in his drawers and his bed still has the drip stand attached to it!

The reason I call what I experienced an 'unwelcome' energy is that somewhere, deep within me, all I really wanted to do was fall apart and cry. I've never been a big crier and so tears are something that have never come easily to me. Perhaps I felt that if I didn't cry, it wasn't real. I thought that crying and grieving went hand in hand. Maybe I wasn't grieving as I should be.

I would get up every morning and get Charlie ready for school, and every morning I would feel grateful that, with our dog in tow, I couldn't go in the playground, therefore I could avoid any contact with other children and parents. My sunglasses became my mask and more often than not I would walk the half hour home again with my eyes full of tears. I couldn't bear to look anybody in the eye. All of a sudden, this was the only routine I had to my days. I remember one morning another mum just came up to me outside the school gates and without saying a word, just silently hugged me. I understood that she didn't know what she could say to me but the fact that my grief had been acknowledged had a huge effect on me. That gesture was bestowed on me on another occasion when I was out shopping. A classroom assistant from Tom's school spotted me and without me having seen her, approached me and did exactly the same thing. These two simple acts were, I think, probably the kindest things anybody had said or done to me since Tom died. There were no words, just empathy and understanding.

Having to cope with other people's reactions is always a terribly hard part of losing your child, and I have spent many hours discussing this topic with bereaved parents at the hospice. I was grateful for the space, together with the reassuring hand of a friend on my arm between me and the person who said to me 'it must have been a blessing in disguise', so as not to retaliate! It is unthinkable that the need to develop a thick skin when you are feeling at your most fragile is almost a necessity when coping with the loss of your child. I have lost count of the number of times I was asked (even at Tom's funeral) whether I would be going back to work. Did people really think that I had had the last nine years off work? Also, no! I didn't want to have another child! All of these reactions only made me feel like the safest place to be at the time was at home, where I didn't have to face the world.

As the first few weeks passed, my energy waned and the only thing I could manage to do in a day was to get Charlie to and from school. The rest of my day would be spent sitting on the sofa trying to make sense of it all. Soon my energy levels dropped drastically and the time spent alone during the day was necessary for me to be able to carry on with some sense of normality when Charlie got home from school again. I never expected the sheer exhaustion that accompanies grieving. To be exhausted from not even doing anything was a totally alien experience for me.

I didn't know what I wanted or what I didn't want. I didn't want to be with people, yet I didn't like being alone. It felt as though I was in a no-win situation. I wanted to be given the opportunity to voice how I was feeling, yet I did not have the words.

I had spent some time during those first few weeks looking for answers to the big question of WHY? I met with doctors who tried to answer my questions and I struggled to accept what I was being told. I needed constant reassurance that I had done all that I possibly could have done to make Tom's life worthwhile and meaningful. I can clearly remember being horribly bothered by reports I had read in the newspaper about medics being criticized and even prosecuted for having administered certain drugs to people in the aftermath of Hurricane Katrina in New Orleans the previous year. There was the suggestion that doctors had been knowingly killing people as acts of compassion using the same drugs I had used to make Tom comfortable at home during his last days. Did this mean I had killed Tom? Thoughts such as these made my days almost unbearable until I had the opportunity to really thrash them out with my GP and Tom's paediatrician, who both assured me that I had done no such thing and that my actions were absolutely right and proper; that I had been brave enough to allow my child to die. One of the doctors from the palliative care team at Great Ormond Street Hospital in London said to me afterwards that I should never underestimate what I had done by allowing Tom to spend his last days at home. It didn't make much sense to me then, but over the years I often think back to that remark with a new-found sense of pride.

Taking this information on board was exhausting, but I can now recognize that it was a crucial part of understanding of the way I was feeling. It was by no means a light-bulb moment—my thoughts and feelings were all over the place and I would have periods of time spent daydreaming about things I could do, places I could go, coupled with agonizing periods of utter despair at why this had happened. I would make decisions only to abandon them at the last moment through a complete lack of motivation. Sometimes, I would be out, and all of a sudden I would decide that I needed to be back at home. I have lost count of the number of times I abandoned shopping plans or left food on a table in my need to make a quick escape. I would find myself trying to do a 'normal' thing such as having a coffee in a coffee shop and then I would be faced with a mother out with an older son, perhaps, and the realization that I would never experience that with Tom was just too much to bear. It was as though I could manage the thoughts in my head but not the actual physical acts required to carry them out.

In Chapter 7, I talk in more detail about when I found situations that were particularly difficult to overcome. One of the most notable, I think, was when I found my sleep was disturbed and when I was feeling unsure as to whether or not I was actually clinically depressed or just experiencing the recognized manifestations of grief. From discussion with my GP, I was led to believe that lack of sleep can lead to depression and vice versa, so this was a tricky road to navigate as I was adamant that I did not want to resort to taking antidepressants or sleeping tablets.

Months later, at a workshop I attended at Helen and Douglas House, I was shown the Dual Process model that Christine Young illustrates later in this chapter. It was as if a misplaced cog had finally found its place in the mess that was my inner turmoil, and things that I had been feeling had been acknowledged and made sense of. The spikiness of the lines criss-crossing the diagram summed up the way my thoughts and actions seemed to change direction on a pinpoint at any given time. Christine will describe later in this chapter about how messy grief is, and this demonstrated it perfectly.

I was struggling with so little meaningful routine to my days. My days with Tom completely revolved around the clock, what with medication, feeds, and changes of position to ensure that his days were spent as comfortably as possible. Out of the blue, an idea of a way to cope with this lack of routine surfaced. It makes me laugh now at the story behind it. I remembered watching the film *About a Boy*, in which Hugh Grant plays a character with a leisurely lifestyle due to royalties earned by his late father. He goes on to explain to a young boy he has befriended unexpectedly about compartmentalizing his day into thirty-minute units just to get through it. Although this fictional situation was about as far from the situation I now found myself in as possible, the thirty-minute strategy was one that I found appealing. I made the decision to change the time to twenty minutes as being less than half an hour it seemed, at the time, more doable. Tentatively, I began to apply it and even if I felt I had just one successful twenty-minute period over the course of the day, I was incredibly pleased with myself.

Over the coming months, I used this strategy increasingly and used it to break up the time where I felt I had sat about for too long with no motivation. I knew that cutting the grass, for example, only took twenty minutes and so I was able to factor in some of the long-neglected things around the house and garden. There have been times since those very early months of my bereavement when I have found myself struggling with situations and I do not hesitate to go back to my twenty-minute plan. I have shared it with other bereaved parents and have been delighted to hear that they have found it to be helpful too. It has become my personal mantra.

A few months ago, when I was contributing to a lecture at St Mary's Hospital in Paddington, London about bereavement, one of the paediatric registrars on the training course asked me what I wished I had known about or been told about. I didn't hesitate in replying that I wish I had been warned that grief *hurt*. Physically hurt. The pain I felt around my heart was real, not a hypothetical pain. It took my breath away and sometimes made me want to fall to my knees. It made me feel sick and as though I couldn't swallow. It made me shake and feel the need to grab on to something to steady me. It sometimes reduced me to tears and at other times to make an involuntary noise, like a gasp. I had no control over it whatsoever. It would come without warning, often in the most inappropriate of places. It was inconvenient and disrespectful. I remember driving to my local shopping centre when an ambulance passed me. It didn't appear to be on an emergency call as there were no blue lights or sirens, but the realization that I had been in so many ambulances with Tom suddenly became too much and I was hit by the full physical force of loss whilst trying to drive my car. Not ideal.

Often these attacks of despair would be accompanied by vivid thoughts about particular scenarios. I can remember describing these to somebody and was told that they were called intrusions. This seemed to sum them up exactly—they intruded into my days and nights and would often lead to a period of intense physical pain. It took many weeks (or more realistically, months) for me to allow 11.15 p.m. on a Saturday night to pass by without being incapacitated by my grief, this being the time that Tom died. It would be *this time two weeks ago… this time three weeks ago*, and so on. I could clearly remember the sounds of his last breaths and it would HURT. I was unable to sleep until that particular time had passed only for the anticipation of it happening the following week to build up along with the harsh fact that another week had passed since Tom's death. I found myself being very aware of the amount of time that had passed since Tom had died. The 29th of each month, for the first year in particular, was a very difficult day to have to anticipate and then live through. It was a constant, painful reminder of time going by without him in my life. Now that I am counting it in years is, I think, a testament to how grief changes over time.

I found that every night when I got into bed and finally turned the light out I would be hit by a huge wave of grief and physical hurt. The silence of the night was deafening, as I had been so used to hearing the hum of Tom's machinery and the soft music that I played in his room at night to settle him. Then on some nights I would wake up suddenly and be sure that I could hear those sounds only for the realization that I had dreamt or imagined them to hit me forcefully.

In those early months spent at home, the internet became virtually my only source of interaction with the world outside my front door. I found games that I could mindlessly play for literally hours, just to pass the time. I discovered The Compassionate Friends website and would spend many, many hours trawling through stories of loss from other people on forums and memorial websites. At first, it helped to make sense of how I was feeling and it helped alleviate the overwhelming feeling of isolation. As weeks and then possibly months went by though, I was beginning to become more and more troubled by the constant thread of negativity to my reading material. I was terrified that I would still be feeling such despair in the years ahead of me. I would read of people who were still not living what I considered to be a valued life many years along in their bereavement. I knew I didn't want to become one of those people. Tom was by far too much a positive part of my life to become the polar opposite.

When I wasn't in front of my computer screen, I found a sense of needing to be outside; to have some contact with the elements and with nature. It made me feel calmer. I began to make plans for my garden. It felt like a safe place to start. It didn't require me having to leave the security and ties I felt to my home. I started to sow seeds and eventually made raised beds to grow vegetables. It taught me a lot about patience. It was impossible to will a seed to germinate and grow; to become strong enough to produce something worthwhile, be it something to eat or something to enjoy the beauty of as a flower. I began to realize that nature was showing me the pace I had to match to get myself to the point where I could live with my loss. It almost seemed incongruous that I should find such a connection with nature whilst living in a London suburb. And there was something that Tom had showed me: that there was much, much more to life than what appeared on the surface.

On Tom's fifteenth birthday, in 2008, I wrote this on my blog:

> *Today Tom would have been 15.*
> *He filled my life with colour and so now I have to find colour elsewhere to get my fix.*
> *Fortunately, my garden is willing to be my colour dealer.*

My garden and my attempts at gardening taught me that patience is indeed a virtue and that things will always continue to grow, and I began to accept that there was no rush to find my new place in this world.

After six months, I received a phone call out of the blue with the tentative offer of doing some voluntary work at Tom's primary school. It took an awful lot of soul-searching to make a decision about whether

I was ready to face a wider world than the one I had chosen to live in for the previous months. Looking back, I can see that it was the first of many small steps I would take in an attempt to reshape my life. It proved to be gentle work, in the school library, categorizing and organizing; reading to small groups of children and encouraging the use of a weekly book bag. The environment was familiar to me and everyone knew my story and, more importantly, knew Tom. There was a memorial to him in the school garden and it felt *right* for me to spend some time in a place where he spent so much of his life.

It was a place where I could avoid the dreaded question—*how many children do you have*? I still have not formulated a satisfactory (to me) response to this enquiry. It is still the one I dread the most. I cannot bear to see the look of horror spread on someone's face if I tell them the truth and equally, I just can't find the comforting words needed to make that other person feel not so awful. I am still adept at avoiding situations where this might arise. Sometimes I felt as though I needed to wear a badge that announced that my child had died to give me an identity and a reason as to why I was behaving the way I was. I attended a service of remembrance at Great Ormond Street Hospital and the chaplain read out this quote from a bereaved mum: 'You do not get over losing a child; you just learn to behave in public'. I would say that sums it up perfectly.

I would read books about grief and losing a child and lines would pop out of the pages and resonate with me to my core:

> 'How will people be able to deal with the person I have become, will become?'
> 'To be forced to be well behaved is torture'

Even in fiction, I found phrases that have stuck with me over the years. The most notable of those being 'grief steers you into rigid self-control'.

Over the course of the following two years, I took up a more regular job at the school and threw myself into long-forgotten hobbies. I found that by making and growing things, my creativity was being nourished again, just as it had been in trying to find ways (sometimes fairly unconventionally!) of making Tom's short life full and happy.

I was encouraged to apply for a teaching degree at university by the staff at the school because they felt I had a lot of experience that could be shared with families of children with special educational needs. I applied and to my complete amazement, I got accepted. It suddenly felt as though I could achieve other things. It felt as though I was succeeding in the mindset of holding on and letting go which was described to me at a spiritual retreat I attended with Helen and Douglas House. Nearing the end of my first year of studying, and having done my first placement, I then decided that teaching was not for me. This coincided with Charlie having difficulties at school and so I left my course. I was determined not to consider this a failure on my part and I now look back on the whole experience with absolutely no regrets, rather with the knowledge that I had succeeded in doing something when I felt that I would never be able to do anything particularly meaningful again.

Eleven months after Tom died, I was invited to my first workshop at Helen and Douglas House. I would say it was one of the most nerve-wracking experiences of my entire life: walking into a room where the only thing any one of those people in there knew was that I had lost a child. It was a complete eye-opener. Here I was, with *real* people who shared my experience; people who would listen to and understand the way I was feeling and were 'qualified' to acknowledge it. Our stories were all different and yet I felt a huge amount of comfort in the simple sharing of our conversations. It opened my eyes to situations that were drastically different from my own and allowed me to feel empathy and compassion. Both were welcome when I had spent so long virtually unable to feel anything other than despair. Suddenly, it felt that by sharing with people who had never even met Tom, it proved to me that my life could continue and be allowed to be shaped by him despite him not being here. I could discuss my feelings of guilt and torment about wanting to move forward without Tom but find comfort in the thought that he was somehow guiding me and willing me to make sense of everything.

I have reaped the rewards of being given the opportunity of joining a bereaved parents group and have attended many workshops that were structured in focusing on different aspects of grief. Once again, I was struck by the fact that such candid emotional opening up was exhausting. I think the first workshop I attended probably took me three days to recover from! They allowed me to embrace the honest and realistic approach I wanted to take with my grief and, at the same time, allow the mask of being completely *fine* that I wore most days, to slip. They gave me the courage to talk about my grief and were certainly the first steps towards taking on the roles that I have played in the last year or so, especially the peer-to-peer support at Helen and Douglas House.

The workshops were attended by parents at several different stages of their grief, and I believe that this is so useful because it allows us to see either how far we have come or that there is a distant hope when your grief is so new and raw. Three years after Tom had died I was asked to participate in a workshop at Helen and Douglas House looking at 'how grief changes over time'. I was the most newly bereaved of the parents on the panel and I have heard that it was one of the most successful workshops that had been held there. It was of huge benefit to me too, as I could take comfort in the words from my fellow members of the panel (one mum was six years post bereavement and the other fourteen years) about what I could perhaps expect to feel in the coming years.

Professional Perspective

Grief combines an often startling range of emotions, which can leave people confused, overwhelmed, and exhausted. You may feel searing pain and sadness, shock, anger, guilt, anxiety, or relief. Initially you will almost certainly feel numb and find the reality of the death hard to take in. Many parents have described it as being like an emotional rollercoaster with unpredictable twists and turns, while for others there is no let up and it is a steady run of overwhelmingly difficult feelings. In my work with bereaved parents the two questions I am most frequently asked are, 'Is this normal?' and 'Am I going mad?'. Typically, the behaviour prompting the questions lies within the range of what is normal and there is no indication of madness, but what these queries highlight is how little most of us know about what to expect in grief and how much it can actually feel like madness. It is often said that grief is a very personal and individual experience; however, it will be shaped by a number of factors. These include whether the death was anticipated or sudden, the relationship with the deceased, previous experiences of loss, and also how much support the bereaved person is receiving or at least perceives him or herself to be receiving. That said, what we have seen at Helen and Douglas House is that there are many aspects of grief, which are shared by the majority of parents, and it is on these that we will focus.

What can we say about parents' experiences of grief? If you take nothing else from this book, take the certain knowledge that people can and do live through it. At Helen and Douglas House we do not see people getting over their grief but, as Tracy talked about in the Introduction, we have seen her, and people like her, learning to live with grief. If you are in the early stages of grief (and that is, of course, a relative term) you will probably find that almost impossible to believe. Certainly grief alters perception, but when you are numb or struggling to focus or frequently overwhelmed by tears it can be extremely hard to see a way through. Borrow from other parents' experience and remind yourself that gradually you will come to a less painful place. What parents describe and what I have seen in practice is that while you do not get over grief, it does change over time. You will not feel this way forever.

Much has been written about the process of grief and loss, but much of the research has been conducted with widows and widowers. To bereaved parents, it sometimes seems as if these explanations don't quite fit and their grief is measured against a standard which does not fully apply. The bereaved generally experience a sense of isolation, and this is heightened for grieving parents, whose experience is outside the norm on so many fronts. For many it is, as Tracy described earlier, the most painful event of their lives. We will take a look at some models of grief and see what they can offer parents in terms of both understanding and managing their bereavement.

Central to much of what we know about grief is 'attachment theory'. This was developed from the work of John Bowlby and when reduced to its simplest form suggests that all social animals form attachments to each other, the purpose of which is to provide safety and security. When that attachment is threatened or destroyed, the reaction is to cry and to search for the lost person. It makes sense that the more intense the attachment, the more intense the reaction, which clearly has implications for parental grief. Based on his work with infants and children, and later applied to the bereaved, Bowlby took the view that grief is an instinctual response to separation, and he and Colin Murray Parkes shared the thinking that in grief we see a pattern of responses to death. This led to the stages and phases approach to grief.

Murray Parkes[1] has written about there being four phases of grief. The first stage is numbness, characterized by feelings of shock, denial, and disbelief. For many parents that numbness is what helps them get through the early days after a death. Feelings of shock and disbelief may be what help you to plan a funeral and, maybe, even speak at it without becoming completely undone. Some parents I have supported have later described this time as being trance or dream like.

The second phase of this model is yearning or pining, characterized by searching, hallucinating, reminiscing, and feelings of anger, guilt and resentment. This phase is sometimes referred to as the 'pangs of grief', where people experience waves of overwhelming emotion, which may well up at any time. In my experience these 'pangs of grief' are very familiar to bereaved parents as is their completely unpredictable nature. Parents are often shocked by the intensity of the emotion and also by their inability to control it when it does break over them. While family members anticipate and try to prepare for the feelings they might have at their child's funeral or on his or her birthday it is the everyday emotions that can overwhelm. One parent, Sally, described a trip to the supermarket where she was completely overwhelmed by the sight of her child's favourite food. For another parent it may be a glimpse of a similar wheelchair or hearing a particular song on the radio. These pangs of grief will leave people exhausted and their unpredictability will sometimes heighten the isolation the bereaved routinely experience as parents choose to spend time alone or at home, rather than risk being overwhelmed at work or in their community.

Within this phase, Murray Parkes describes a component of fear and insecurity as people face a new world without the special person, who may have made them feel valued. There is a physiological aspect to this, too, and people often experience physical symptoms of severe anxiety—a knotted stomach, inability to concentrate etc. The physical nature of grief can be a complete surprise. Martin, whose toddler son had recently died, told me 'I had no idea how physical grief would be'. He described a pain around his heart, as Tracy does, too, as being with him fairly constantly. He was also unprepared for how exhausting grieving was. He reported that getting through a day without his son took so much more energy than when his son was alive and needing constant care. Sarah, two of whose daughters had died, was also unprepared for the physical impact. She reflected that it took her close to a couple of years to get back to her normal energy levels and during that time she noticed that she was much more susceptible to any viruses which were going around.

Murray Parkes's third phase is one of disorganization and despair, and is characterized by anxiety, loneliness, ambivalence, fear, hopelessness, and helplessness. Despair comes from the realization that the person who has died will not return. His fourth phase is one of reorganization and recovery, and in this stage the bereaved person begins to re-involve him or herself in life and gain a new identity. This can also require detaching from the dead person and moving on.

As you can see from some of the examples, bereaved parents can relate to much of what is described here. There are two components, however, that do not sit right with what bereaved parents tell us.

The first is that, although Murray Parkes has said that people can move back and forth between the phases, this model has been assimilated into popular culture with the understanding that grief is a journey through the four phases; a neat little package that moves in a linear progression from numbness to moving on; and that it has a time line of around twelve months. Anyone who has been bereaved is aware that there is nothing neat or orderly about grief. It is messy and unpredictable and much more like snakes and ladders than a straight run through the four phases. Further, bereaved parents would strongly dispute that twelve months come even close to being enough time to work through their grief. In fact, many would say that the second year is messier and more painful than the first.

By far the bigger problem for parents, though, is the idea of moving on. The notion of severing links with your child who has died and building a new life creates a dissonance for parents. They want to find ways not to separate from the child but to actually integrate them into this new uncertain existence, which has been forced upon them.

Let's take a look now at two different explanations of grief, one of which acknowledges the less than linear shape that grieving can take (Stroebe and Schut) while the other focuses on parents maintaining, rather than severing the connection with their child (Klass).

The easiest way to describe Margaret Stroebe and Henk Schut's model of grief[2] is with a diagram (Fig. 1.1).

Stroebe and Schut see grief as a dual process consisting of two main responses, one of which is loss-oriented and the other restoration-oriented. Simply put, the left-hand side of the diagram, focusing on loss, is about confronting the emotions of grief and its intensity. The restoration side allows us to avoid grief by keeping busy and getting on with things. Central to this model, though, is the idea of oscillation. The lines moving backwards and forwards between the two sides represent the shifting between feeling distraught at the loss in one moment and in the next coping with the necessities of life, whether that is maintaining structure for a surviving child or talking with a funeral director.

Movement between the two sides allows us to both confront the loss and be distracted from it. Expressing and experiencing feelings of loss twenty-four hours a day would be totally exhausting. This would also

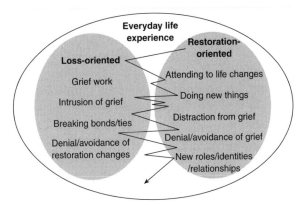

Fig. 1.1 A dual process model for coping with loss. Reproduced from Stroebe and Schut[2] with permission of the Taylor and Francis Group, http://www.informaworld.com.

be true for anyone trying to constantly distract themselves from the painful feelings of loss, so the movement between the two may actually be helpful and healthy. When we have talked about this model at parent groups or workshops it has struck a chord with many participants, there being a general recognition that the oscillation can take place not just over the course of a day, but in much shorter periods of time. The feeling of parents was that in describing grief as being neither static nor linear, Stroebe and Schut capture the messiness of grief we talked about earlier and it has helped parents make sense of their own experience. This model also allows for changes over longer periods of time. In the early days of bereavement there may be a greater concentration of energy focusing on the loss, but as time goes on it may become more restoration-oriented.

Let's now look at the challenge for parents of severing the bond with their child and moving on, as they are frequently encouraged and expected to do. Dennis Klass, an American academic, has worked over many years with bereaved parents, involved with 'Compassionate Friends', a self-help group specifically for parents, who have experienced the loss of a son or daughter. He is a proponent of the idea of continuing bonds.[3]

Central to Klass's thinking and observations is the idea that the resolution of grief involves a continuing bond, which the survivor maintains with the deceased. The purpose of grief is not about breaking a connection with the child and moving on with life, but the bond may be transformed from something painful to something which may give solace and inspiration. For much of the twentieth century a bond with the deceased was viewed as symptomatic of psychological problems and 'unresolved grief'. Bereaved parents were perhaps particularly vulnerable to this labelling or pathologizing, but Klass, in his extensive work with this group, has given us a new interpretation of it which has come directly from the parents themselves. As well as giving us a time line of at least three to four years for parents to develop a new equilibrium, which is secure enough for them to trust, the bereaved parents have also developed a language, which they use to locate themselves and others in this process: they are 'Newly bereaved', 'Into their grief', 'Well along in their grief', and 'Resolved as much as it will be'.

(1) *Newly bereaved.* For parents, their child's death is experienced as an awful truth that seems unreal, and it is very important for them to share that loss with others. Frequently though, parents experience a lack of communal understanding: people will not mention the child or will suggest, for example, that a new baby might replace him or her. When the child dies, it seems to parents as if their lives have stopped, while other people's lives continue and their own sense of isolation can be bitter. Extended family and the wider community struggle with the notion that the child is dead and yet the parent is still bonded to the child. Klass has found that this time of being newly bereaved roughly corresponds to the first year after the child has died.

(2) *Into their grief.* As parents move into this phase Klass suggests that the complexity of the parental bond with the dead child becomes expressed in the complexity of the parents' grief. He writes about the shared bonds, which develop in support groups, in which the children who have died become very much part of that community. Pain is shared, as are ways of relieving that pain. This is also something which we have seen time and again in support groups at Helen and Douglas House. In coming together with others in a similar situation, parents feel understood, less

isolated, and in the sharing of the group they find their experience can be helpful to the others.

(3) *Well along in their grief.* As parents begin to find a new equilibrium they hold the child differently in their minds, and in Klass's experience this is formulated in terms of holding on and letting go. He suggests that parents may be able to let go of the pain and hold on to the energy and love that were in the living child. In the context of a supportive group of grieving parents the children are by now the heart and soul of the group. The individual bond the parent has with the child is now shared with the group.

(4) *Resolved as much as it will be.* One of Klass's parents says, 'You don't get over your grief, but it doesn't stay the same'. At this point the message that parents can give to more recently bereaved parents is that it will always hurt, but it will not hurt the way it does now. The bonds which parents have with their children are complex, so transforming them is a long and exhausting process; however, parents do find that they are able to do this. Sometimes they may have paradoxical feelings about completing that particular process of grief. One recently bereaved Helen and Douglas House father, who listened to another parent talking about how she no longer hurt the way she had previously, responded that he did not want to stop hurting. In his mind his pain was a link to his son, which he was not prepared to relinquish. Accepting that the pain has diminished can be a loss in itself.

Part of the resolution of grief is making the pain count for something, or put another way, making the parent's life, especially the experience of their child's life and death, count for something. One way for parents to make their lives count seems to be to help others. This can take many forms, from supporting other bereaved families to raising funds to provide services or to fund research.

Klass's conclusion is that the end of grief is not when the bond with the child is severed, but rather when the child is integrated into the parents' lives in a different way from when the child was alive. This depiction of how parents experience grief closely matches what we see in our work with families at Helen and Douglas House. The child continues to be a significant part of parents' lives, but in a positive and less painful way.

These theories can be helpful, but what of the day-to-day experience of grief? Without doubt it will impact every aspect of your life. It is a multi-dimensional process and you will see and feel its effect on your emotional, cognitive, spiritual, physical, and sexual self. We have previously mentioned parents being overwhelmed by tears and sadness when they least expect it. You may also feel angry at the whole world or at things that simply are not that important. There may be regrets and guilt about what you might have done differently and a sense of injustice when you look at other intact families. Do not be surprised if somewhere in the mix you feel some relief. One parent, Robert, shared in a group that this was one of his first reactions to the death of his son. The relief was followed by some brief thoughts about the life that he and his wife and daughters would now be able to have, unrestricted by care needs, before being swiftly overtaken by guilt. The full range of feelings may come thick and fast. Sometimes it is hard to separate out the emotions and all you may be aware of is how awful it feels.

Grief may change your thoughts and behaviour, too. Some parents struggle to erase memories of their child's last days or hours while happier memories elude them. Sometimes the activities you once loved may just seem too much to think about or you may find yourself strongly driven by an enormous need to keep busy. The distraction provided by racing around and never staying still can keep painful thoughts and memories at bay for a short time, but they usually find their way to the surface at some point.

Grief can also affect your concentration. Parents repeatedly find that their mind wanders or they simply cannot retain information in the way they used to do. If you find yourself reading the same page or paragraph over and over again and still not taking it in, don't panic. It is likely that a combination of fatigue and stress are at the heart of this. Bernadine Cimprich of the University of Michigan has researched this in breast cancer patients, but her findings have been generalized to include a broader population. Her work has shown that spending time in nature, at least twenty minutes a day, can improve cognitive functioning, so a short walk or time spent in the garden may help you take in information and also retain it. You can read what she has to say on this by following this web link: http://www.med.umich.edu/cancer/living/natures-medicine.html.

We talked earlier about the physical nature of grief and how tiring it is. Perhaps what is most useful to say at this point is that you will benefit from acknowledging the limitations that exhaustion places on you and pacing yourself accordingly. Factor fatigue into your schedule and lower your expectations of yourself. While we all benefit from sufficient rest and a balanced diet, it is probably of especial value when you are grieving. Sometimes family members and friends do not know how to give emotional support, but may offer help with practical things. Accept all offers—don't refuse a meal being provided or the garden being done. Conserve the energy you have for the things you really want or need to do.

Losing a child can also impact on sexuality, and partners may not always see this in the same way. Grief may make physical intimacy increasingly important as it can create closeness, a sense of connectedness and perhaps provide temporary distraction from the pain of loss. On the other hand it can reinforce the loss by reminding a parent of their child's conception and for a couple whose son or daughter has had a genetic condition, this can resonate even more strongly. Some parents simply feel that sex is inappropriate at this time when you may ask yourself how you can enjoy something pleasurable when your child has died. In Chapter 4 we will look in more detail at the impact of grief on couples. For now the critical thing to say is talk with your partner about what is going on between you and help each other understand what each of you is thinking and feeling. Silence or lack of response may be easily misinterpreted and can add to the isolation each of you may be feeling. As with most relationship issues, communication is key.

At the beginning of this chapter we raised the question of what is normal in grief and what might feel like madness. Most of what people experience lies somewhere between the two, but you may have concerns which could benefit from discussion with a professional. There is a point at which some bereaved parents wonder if they are clinically depressed. We know that grief changes mood and depletes energy. It would not be difficult to confuse the sadness of grief with clinical depression, so we need to be able to differentiate between the two. David Kissane in *Family Focused Grief Therapy*[4] suggests that grieving people still have the ability to respond to joyful experiences. By contrast, depressed people lose this ability. So how can you tell for yourself? You may need help with this. If you think that you may be clinically depressed it would be a good idea to go and talk with your GP. He or she will be able to determine that with you. A conversation with your GP is essential if you have thoughts of harming yourself.

I have heard parents at different points in their grief express a desire to be with their child. This might come from a place of feeling that they need to care for him or her or from an intense longing to see or touch them one more time. I know of parents who have worried about the child being alone. If you find that you are moving beyond a desire or longing to be with your son or daughter to actually having a plan to hurt yourself and the means to carry it out then you must speak with your GP immediately.

It is normal for grief to hurt and for it to disrupt sleep, but when feelings become too difficult or sleep so disturbed that it is hard to function, you may think about medication. Discussion of this with parents suggests to me that people are divided into camps on this; a group who would never consider medication and another group who are cautiously curious. There can be risks either way. Sometimes it can be helpful to ask parents in the first group if they would refuse medication for high blood pressure or diabetes. The answer to that question is generally 'no'. This, of course, speaks volumes about how we view physical and mental health and their associated treatments. Medication for a physical condition is viewed as essential, while for an emotional condition it is frequently viewed as denoting weakness, or raises apprehensions about addiction. I have often heard parents talk about having to be strong and just get through this. Sometimes, though, strength lies in challenging a long-held belief and accepting help and support, whether that help comes in the form of a trusted friend or medication.

From the work I have done with families, my impression is that many parents live with their grief without the use of any medication. However, grief sometimes becomes an obstacle that prevents parents functioning in the way that they need and want to. Here, prescribed medication may make a difference. It can help a parent obtain the sleep he or she needs to face the day ahead or make it more likely that they will be available for their surviving children. A pill will not deal with the underlying emotional issues, but by helping with the symptoms it can be an effective tool in getting you to a place where you can begin to look at the sadness, anger, or guilt that is at the root cause of your distress.

Medication is only one response to the pain of grief. Many parents are comforted by family, friends or spiritual beliefs. As Klass's research shows, and practice at Helen and Douglas House confirms, there can also be huge benefit to parents in meeting with others who are also grieving. Talking with and listening to others facing similar difficulties will confirm that you are not the only person feeling the way you do. It will help you feel less isolated and also answer those questions in your head about whether your grief is normal or whether you are going mad. If your sense is that family or colleagues at work have no clue about what you are faced with, a support group may be the place where you will feel understood.

Try to be open-minded about all kinds of support. Sometimes parents tell me that they do not need a group or want to see their GP about medication as they have never needed anything like that before. That may well be true, but the likelihood is that you have never confronted grief like this before, either.

As well as your internal feelings or state of mind, there is also the issue of dealing with the external world. What can you expect from family, friends, co-workers etc.? In the best of circumstances they will be there for you, but it appears that parents are on the receiving end of responses which run the gamut. You will most likely encounter marvellous kindness and understanding, alongside some examples of breath-taking insensitivity. You will be offered help and you will be avoided. Some people will acknowledge your loss and others will completely ignore it. You may find that while you have no idea or concept of how long you will grieve for, others will have firm views about how long it should take. Usually their expectation is that it will be of a shorter duration than is realistic. Other people's responses to your loss and how to handle them are tackled in Chapters 5 and 7, but for now know that alongside those who really come through, not everyone will be there for you in the way you might like. It is not personal, however how much it may feel that it is. Every bereaved parent has been on the receiving end of crass or insensitive comments, just as they have all experienced astonishing acts of support and generosity.

Things to Remember

Your experience of grief will be unique, but it may be helpful to be aware of these general points:

- Grief is not an orderly process. It will affect every aspect of your life—cognitive, physical, emotional, sexual, spiritual, and social

- It will take longer than you (and the people around you) think to feel life has any order or stability

- Grieving consumes an enormous amount of energy, so accept offers of help and conserve your strength for what is important

- Keep an open mind about what or who might help you—family, friends, a support group, counselling, or possibly medication

- Other parents before you have lived through this. Hard as it is to believe, you will too

References

1. Parkes, C.M. (1996) *Bereavement: studies of grief in adult life*, 3rd edn. Penguin, London.

2. Stroebe, M. and Schut, H. (1999) The dual process model of coping with bereavement: rationale and description. *Death Studies*, **23**, 197–224.

3. Klass, D. (1996) The deceased child in the psychic and social worlds of bereaved parents during the resolution of grief. In: *Continuing bonds: new understandings of grief* (ed. D. Klass, P.R. Silverman, and S.L. Nickman), pp. 199–216. Taylor and Francis, London.

4. Kissane, D.W. and Bloch, S. (2002) *Family focused grief therapy: a model of family-centred care during palliative care and bereavement*. Open University Press, Buckingham.

Your Notes

Chapter 2

Secondary losses

Parent's Perspective

One of the hardest things to come to terms with when your child dies is the loss of your whole way of life as you know it. There are many, many secondary losses that are never, at least in my experience, considered beforehand. I suppose that the knowledge that you are going to lose your child is so huge that it is impossible to contemplate anything more than the loss of life.

For me, the most profound secondary loss was that of having such an empty life after Tom died. Having been so surrounded and supported by a vast team of professionals who guided me through virtually all of Tom's needs, it was as though somebody had simply erased them all from my existence. For many years, my diary had been filled with all manner of appointments and meetings that allowed Tom to live comfortably with me at home. I had a regular team of carers who felt like part of the family and I had doctors and other medical professionals with whom I could share my worries. I had not gone back to work since having Charlie, and so my full-time job became that of a stay-at-home mum with the added pressures and responsibilities of having such a dependent child as well as a very young one. It felt as if the multidisciplinary team had become my colleagues and they were often my only source of adult conversation. It was always extremely important to me to feel as though I was part of 'Team Tom', as I liked to think of it, and so after he died it felt as though the team had moved on without me and I was left at the headquarters alone, with no purpose.

I considered myself lucky to be so comfortable as part of this team and I believe that it was the relationships that I always strived to build with the people who were involved in our life that made a massive difference to the way my opinions and needs were dealt with. I became Tom's advocate and tried to include all aspects of his well-being in his care and treatment—emotionally, mentally, and physically. I didn't want his individuality compromised by textbook treatment. Another bereaved parent who I have spent time with likened it to being made redundant but left in an empty office.

Slowly, after the frantic funeral planning, more and more people faded from view and it wasn't long before I felt that not only was I living in a shell of a house but a shell of a life too. I was still able to take care of Charlie and the basic day-to-day parts of my own life but it seemed that the most important part had disappeared with Tom too: that was my own role and identity. I felt abandoned.

It felt almost perverse to miss going to the hospital regularly, or welcoming my GP into my home on a fortnightly basis. I missed drawing up medicine and even washing up syringes. I missed the routine that had become integral to our life. It felt as though nothing had any direction or meaning anymore; that nothing was urgent. I wasn't used to having more time than I knew what to do with.

During Tom's life I always felt well supported by my team, and afterwards my life felt very tenuous and fragile. I didn't have the reassurance from them that it was all right because I felt so devastated. Whereas I'd always had guidance, I was now floundering in an unknown space that I couldn't identify with.

In the lead up to the first Christmas without Tom, I recall asking Charlie how he would like Christmas to be that year. He didn't hesitate in replying that he wanted it to be the same as all the previous years—the big family Christmas at our house with all the trimmings. I baulked on the inside at the very thought but I was struck by the realization that I would hate Charlie to feel that he'd lost his mother, in a sense, as well as his brother. I had always delighted in entertaining our family, and loved going to all the effort to make occasions such as Christmas or Easter or birthdays memorable. Would Charlie think that I didn't consider he was worth making an effort for? The whole situation felt very complicated because as much as I really couldn't face making such a big effort because of the hole that I felt not having Tom there had created, I also felt that Charlie had the absolute right to a memorable childhood too. I was worried that, at the age of ten,

Charlie had, because of losing Tom, lost some of the innocence of his childhood already. He had had to face very real things very early on. He had had to experience the worst and it broke my heart to watch him being so brave every day to protect me.

Charlie does not have any memory of Tom before he became ill because he was only ten months old when it happened. He grew up in the midst of a very different life from the one that his peers would be living. At a very young age, he became knowledgeable in many aspects of Tom's care and requirements. I can remember overhearing him once telling one of the carers '*actually*, we use TWO mouth swabs for Tom's oral care, not ONE'. I think he was about 3 years old and I smiled at the stunned silence of the carer as we caught each other's eye! So, he obviously didn't miss a trick. This particular carer was a nurse with over twenty-five years' experience, and I also delighted in hearing him tell her that we flushed Tom's gastrostomy tube with 20 ml of water, not 10 ml! It does feel, to some degree, that I lost a part of Charlie's childhood as well as my role as his mother because of Tom becoming ill. It felt compromised. Charlie had both his first and second birthday parties in hospital playrooms rather than at home.

I have taken part in many discussions about how remaining siblings become part of the secondary losses that you come to experience when you lose your child. I felt very strongly that Charlie's identity had also been lost as a sibling—he was now an only child and that wasn't how it was meant to be. I hadn't chosen to have only one child and it felt as though I had lost the experience of watching my children grow up together and do the things that brothers are expected to do with one another. To look out for each other, and fight and argue as well as protect and love each other. Not only had I lost my identity as Tom's carer and advocate, but also I had lost the role of being a mother to boys in the plural.

One of the hardest parts of supporting some of the bereaved parents I have met has been if they have lost their only child. They feel that they are no longer a parent. It has been as though they have been stripped of absolutely every identity they ever possessed. It has been extraordinarily difficult to have been told that it is all right for me because I have still got Charlie. It has shown me just how personal and complicated grief is.

I once made a book for Charlie containing some photographs of him and Tom together over the years. I found a quote on the internet that I used on the first page that said 'it takes two boys to make one brother'. This seemed to sum up exactly how I felt about Charlie's role then. I will talk about this book more in Chapter 10, Creating memories.

It started to dawn on me that, with hindsight, I had lost much of Charlie's early years as a direct consequence of Tom becoming ill, as Tom more often than not had to be the priority in the sense of need: most things revolved around him. While Tom was alive, I had never really given much thought to this as I was so immersed in the life we had, but after he died I began to realize that there were many other losses that I would be facing, and some of them were from the past but were going to have to be faced now. My grief for Tom was going to have to include a whole lot of other issues that had gone before. I would never have realized how sad I would find it having my youngest child doing the things that my eldest child never had the chance to. This has been a particularly strong emotion as Charlie has grown into a teenager and begins to tentatively plan his future.

As I became stronger emotionally, it felt like I had been given a chance to face up to and work through many things that I had not had the time to deal with previously. I have had the opportunity to talk to the bereavement team, other bereaved parents, and a counsellor from my GP's surgery. I have dissected aspects of my failed marriage, my relationship with my extended family, and my place in my social circle.

In the early days of bereavement, a numbness took over that I talked about in the previous chapter. This inevitably led to a loss of confidence because I felt a growing sense of isolation. The less I went out or spoke to people, the less I felt able to do it. The impact of losing Tom had left me feeling so very vulnerable, and I would experience panic attacks when I tried to do seemingly normal social activities such as going out for dinner with friends. Like the intrusions I talked of in the previous chapter, they would happen at the most inconvenient of times and did nothing to help me find the confidence to try and take up some semblance of life again. I would become nauseous and uncomfortable, with the need to be in the fresh air but also to be away from everybody. My heart would race, and it felt like I had to concentrate even on breathing. I would become scared of being on my own; scared of not being able to cope; scared of worrying Charlie; scared of anyone seeing me not coping. My pride was very important to me. I was a coper. A strong person. I couldn't bear people to see me at my most fragile and I could barely look anyone in the eye.

I think I developed a method for self-protection by identifying certain situations that I knew could be potentially upsetting, and this lack of confidence contributed to me choosing to avoid them.

Paradoxically, as time passed, it became noticeable that this loss of confidence also gave way to what felt like a loss of fear. There have been times when I have felt that I am quite invincible, that nothing can hurt me now because the worst had already happened. This feeling came over me once in a very unpleasant situation. My dad had a heart attack while waiting for bypass surgery and I rushed to my parents' house to find him being treated in the ambulance with the paramedic and ambulance crew. Sitting beside him I had the most unwelcome feeling of acquiescence, as though it was bad, but not that bad, because Tom had died and nothing could be as bad as that. I was shocked to the core at the intensity of this feeling and it made me feel uncomfortable and guilty. I worried that this lack of fear had made me an awful person.

It is not a wholly negative feeling though. I look at my life now and feel it has focus to it because I have not been afraid to try things. I have always been an optimistic person, and this optimism, coupled with the lack of fear, has opened up many new doors for me in an effort to regain some definition to my life. As I said in the Introduction, I am now living with my grief and it has allowed me take interest in new things and see them with, what feels like, a different pair of eyes. I have a strong need to take notice of the detail of everything and so have become increasingly keen on photography to try to capture as much as I can as a permanent record. I have made my macro lens my best friend because it allows me to see the detail close up. I am particularly keen on photographing the intricate parts of flowers. It is as though I have this need to see what it is that is the core of something. I like to think that Tom is at the very core of me and will always remain so. I was delighted to discover that another bereaved mum who I met at a workshop had exactly the same need. It was as though we shared the same obsession! It is quirky little connections like this that I have found to be welcome positives in such a devastating experience.

The process of regaining a positive identity has been very much a trial and error undertaking and I feel as though I have dipped my toes into many things to find out what it is that will restore my equilibrium. I still do not know where I am ultimately going or who I am going to be, but I do feel determined to embrace the journey rather than worry over the end destination.

Professional Perspective

In the wake of a son's or daughter's death, parents are typically unprepared for the subsequent erosion of the life they have known. You will increasingly become aware of many things which have ended, with no indication, or perhaps desire, for new beginnings. You may feel that not only have you lost your son or daughter, but that you have also lost much of your world. What Tracy has described is in no way unique to her situation, but is shared in different ways by most bereaved parents. There is no question that the death of a son or daughter brings huge additional and usually unexpected losses. This may be especially true in families where the child has had a long-term illness or condition, but it equally applies in situations of sudden death. While, as parents, we may joke or complain about our children's lives taking over our own, few of us truly realize the extent of the web woven around us by our children's needs, which contribute to the routine and structure of our daily life. It is not until it is suddenly blown away that its absence is palpable and we recognize its significance.

Following the death of a child the rhythm of normal life is completely disrupted. Whether your schedule as a parent involved managing carers and doctors' appointments or making sure you got your child to school or college, the pattern will be wiped out overnight. For the typical Helen and Douglas House family—if such a thing exists— long-term caring often means that one or both parents will have given up work outside of the family home to focus on caring for their child. As a result of this, friendships and other relationships can be difficult to maintain, to the point that sometimes the army of carers rotating through the house become the primary link with the outside world and in some cases the family's main social contact. Some agencies and services continue to be involved with the family for a short time after the child has died, but frequently that relationship ends with the child's death, or within a few days of it. Equipment may swiftly be removed from the home and if the family has a mobility vehicle that too will have to be returned sooner than imagined. Your regular visits to the children's hospital or hospice will also become a thing of the past.

This means that the enormous loss of a beloved son or daughter is compounded by the loss of the associated structure and routine which his or her life required, as well as the loss of the people involved in providing it. One parent described this experience as a 'deafening silence'. In times of crisis many of us fall back on the routine and familiar to help pull us through, but parents in the midst of their grief find that the routine and familiar have disappeared, too. Moreover, they are challenged to rebuild a life for themselves at a time when their emotional and physical resources are seriously depleted and often when self-confidence is at a very low point.

The loss of the hands-on parenting of your child, in combination with the absence of your usual plans for your day, may leave you questioning your identity and your existence. If you have been wondering who you are now, when you are no longer parenting your child, you are not alone. These questions usually surface alongside others about what you will do with your life. If it is your only child who has died, you may well be asking yourself if you are, in fact, still a parent at all, even if you know in your heart that ultimately you will always be that. Parents recognize fairly early on that even though their child is physically absent, they are still his or her parents and will continue to be so. The child continues to be a significant part of the family mentally, emotionally, or spiritually. One Helen and Douglas House couple whose only son died understood this, but still ached for the real hands-on parenting they no longer carried out. The part of their social life which came from being parents of a toddler also became uncertain territory. Would the other parents still welcome them as part of their group and could the bereaved parents cope with being around their son's playmates? Would it be too painful to watch others with their children, when their own parenting role was now largely invisible?

Expect to be fazed by questions about whether you have children or how many you have. They make the awful truth real and stir anxiety about how others will respond to your answer. They also highlight the questioning that goes on in your own mind. How do you explain your role and identity now that your child is no longer physically present? The question of role and identity is not easily resolved, but it does become clearer and more settled as time passes. You should, however, anticipate a spell of not quite knowing who you are and of questioning the meaning and value of what you are doing. And it is not just parental identity that is shaken, but the concept of family too. I have heard from many parents, struggling to reshape family life in a group that is now three instead of four, that this is just not how it was meant to be. Siblings have to grapple with this, too, as they adjust to being an only child or question what their new place is in the family order. What does it mean for a child when their older sibling dies at age twelve and they surpass them, by turning thirteen? One sibling has recently talked about not wanting to reach that age where she will technically become older than her sister.

Aside from its composition, perceptions of the family may change too. Numerous families have commented on feeling that they are no longer 'special'. Parents of children with a life-limiting or terminal condition are often admired for how well they manage the demands of care. They are seen as admirable or coping in a way that others cannot imagine. The admiration may well disappear when the child dies, and it is sometimes replaced by pity. The sense of being special is lost. This is not limited to those caring for a sick child. One of the secondary losses for parents of twins, one of whom died very suddenly, was of a similar nature: Lynn and Steve had felt great pride in parenting twins and enjoyed the special nature of their two little boys, but felt that this was also lost to them when Lucas suddenly died. Absorbed in the day-to-day routine of parenting, few of us are aware of the hopes and dreams we have for our children and for our families. When a child dies, parents lose the expectations they had for their child as well as their hopes about future family life or the relationship the child might have shared with his or her siblings.

In the early days of grief, a lot of parents comment on how hard it is to get up and face the day, whether from lack of structure or a feeling that life lacks purpose. Alan struggled to find any point in getting up and going to work, and what I frequently hear from parents is that for many of them the preferred option would be to stay in bed, buried under the duvet. The thing that amazes me is how infrequently that happens. Parents somehow find the drive to keep going, even in the most awful of circumstances. Some have found it helpful to break the day down into smaller units of time. Tracy has explained her 'twenty-minute rule', which was simply to select a task and plan to do it for twenty minutes, at the end of which you can choose to stop or to carry on. Other parents have developed their own variations of this, and so begin to create structure by building on very small tasks or goals. Alan, the dad mentioned above, has built time into his working day during which he can to go to his daughter's grave. He has also managed to find other points in the day when he can take a little bit of time out if he needs to do so. While this does not resolve the bigger problem of meaning or purpose, it allows him to anchor his day by building into it something of significance to him.

I think that the hardest part of facing the void in so many areas of life is the anxiety it produces and the accompanying uncertainty about how long it might last. What parents gradually find is that while nothing will fill the place of their child, other routines and structures do gradually evolve which help them towards a life that is still meaningful. It is important to allow things to happen at your own pace. Well-meaning friends and family will probably encourage you to go out and do things or go back to work. If that feels right, do it, but don't be pressured into being busy just to make others feel better. Allow yourself to be yourself and to choose the direction in which you want to go. In Chapter 1 we talked about how we might respond to grief were it a physical illness rather than an assault on the emotions. Similarly, had you been seriously ill or undergone major surgery, you would be very careful about pacing yourself back into everyday life. Anna, a bereaved mother, was terribly anxious that she had forever lost her incredible drive and motivation which had been major assets in advocating for her son's care while he was alive. She was terrified by her lack of energy and felt she should be doing more to put her life back on track. Now, almost a year on, she sees both the energy and drive gradually returning. It is no longer being used for her son's life, but is helping her reshape both her own life and that of her family.

Sometimes, when thinking about what to do next, parents are drawn to finding work as carers or in a field related to their son's or daughter's illness. They often talk about wanting to help other families in a situation similar to their own experience. That is true for siblings, too. At Helen and Douglas House we have seen siblings go to medical school or train to be nurses as a direct result of what has happened to their brother or sister. Wanting to help other families is understandable, but it needs to be approached with caution. Many parents and siblings are experts at delivering care and would be an asset in a range of settings, but there can be an emotional cost to this. Supporting a child or family like your own can touch on some very raw emotions, especially in the first year or two following your bereavement. Taking up a caring career while you are still coming to terms with your own child's death may make grieving more difficult or prolong it. If it is an option in which you are seriously interested, give yourself time to come to terms with your own grief before embarking on it.

Similarly if you have a job or volunteering role to which you may return, think carefully about whether it is a job you will still be able to do, or what support you might need to make it so. Some parents find work a welcome distraction from grief, while others resent the time and energy it takes. Your focus and concentration will not be as sharp as they were and that can impact upon your performance. The nature of the work is critical, too. One Helen and Douglas House parent, Tina, really enjoyed her job in the emergency services. However, when she went back to work about six months after her daughter Jordie had died, the frequent contact with trauma and death compounded her grief and she realized that at least for the time being she could not continue to do that kind of work. The context of Tina's grief was different from that of most parents in that she had earlier been bereaved of her son, Jack, and was in effect grieving for two children. What is similar to other parents' experience though, is the realization that a job which was manageable before may now be more difficult. If you encounter this, or a similar problem, talk with your line manager, human resources department, or occupational health service. Sometimes companies can accommodate shifts in roles or temporary changes to work schedules etc. It is really important that in thinking about future roles you look at the skills you have, but also at what the emotional demands of a particular job might be.

If you are reading this chapter as a parent anticipating the death of your child I cannot stress how important it is that you try to keep some part of your own life going. I know how hard it is to find any time for yourself and how much harder it can be to justify such time, but it is something which will help you both in caring for your son or daughter now and in managing your grief in the future. Dr Jan Aldridge writes eloquently about this in *Living With a Seriously Ill Child*[1] and I recommend it to you.

If you are a bereaved parent, remember that what feels like a gaping hole will not remain forever. A different life will eventually develop around the void, even if it does not fill it. Lois Tonkin, a New Zealand grief counsellor, has written about a bereaved mum who described her grief as follows. Her child had died some years before and at that time her grief had totally consumed her, filling every part of her life. Her expectation was that the grief would shrink and become encapsulated in her life in a small and manageable way. But what happened was different. The grief stayed as it was and her life grew around it. There were times when she felt the grief intensely, but more and more she was able to live in the life around it (Fig. 2.1).

Nothing will either take or fill the place your child has had in your life but, like the mother who inspired Tonkin's diagram, you will rebuild a life around the loss; one which will ultimately have meaning and purpose.

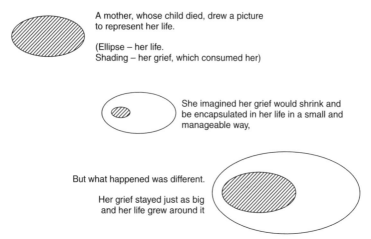

A mother, whose child died, drew a picture to represent her life.

(Ellipse – her life.
Shading – her grief, which consumed her)

She imagined her grief would shrink and be encapsulated in her life in a small and manageable way,

But what happened was different.

Her grief stayed just as big and her life grew around it

Fig. 2.1 The Tonkin model of growing around grief. Reproduced from Tonkin[2] with permission of the Taylor & Francis Group, http://www.informaworld.com.

Things to Remember

- You may feel that you have lost not only your child, but your world too
- You may question your identity
- You may reassess work and life priorities
- You may struggle without the previous structure and routine
- You will have to adjust to the changed family composition

Reference

1. Aldridge, J. (2007) *Living with a seriously ill child*. Sheldon Press, London.
2. Tonkin, L. (1996) Growing around grief — another way of looking at grief and recovery. *Bereavement Care*, **15**, 10, with permission of the Taylor & Francis Group, http://www.informaworld.com.

Your Notes

Chapter 3

Supporting surviving children

Parent's Perspective

In October 2005, seven months before Tom died, he was taken ill at school and rushed into hospital. During this stay, which lasted for ten days due to another chest infection, I had what I will always consider *the conversation* with his paediatrician. I knew that Tom's life was limited and I knew that his chest was becoming weaker and weaker. I made the decision to voice my fears to the doctor and ask about what I needed to know about him dying. At this time one of my overwhelming concerns was about how Charlie would react and cope with such news. As was my usual practice, I was determined to glean as much information as possible for my coping mechanisms to kick in.

Fortunately, the doctor offered to talk to Charlie for me, and this felt like a lifeline as I just didn't feel as though I was equipped to deal with the situation on my own. I think I felt that I had invested so much time in trying to ensure that Charlie didn't ever have to worry about Tom and all his obvious disabilities and illnesses, that I felt guilty about then dropping this bombshell, as I am convinced that Charlie would not, at his young age, ever have considered that this could happen.

We made an appointment and I took Charlie to the ward in the hospital that was all too familiar. We sat in the teenagers' sitting room and I had to sit and watch as Charlie was told that because of Tom's illness from many years ago and the subsequent disabilities and difficulties he had endured since, his body was becoming tired and worn out. Charlie sat there beside me and allowed this information to be so eloquently given to him. Instinctively I could tell that all the time his thoughts were about me. When he was asked if he'd like to ask any questions, he declined. I wasn't wholly surprised at this because he was always such an accepting child when it came to facing anything that concerned his brother. He had never once questioned why any of this should happen to either Tom or himself. To see him acting so stoically made my heart ache. The level of maturity and self-control that Charlie always displayed was a bittersweet thing for me to witness. I always worried that he mirrored the behaviour I was guilty of: *always* coping, *always* remaining strong and focused. It almost seemed unnatural in one so young.

In the days leading up to Tom's death my thoughts, again, were focused on Charlie just as much as they were on Tom. I knew that my wish to have Tom comfortable at home could lead to things that would be extremely traumatic for Charlie to witness. At the time, Charlie was a Cub Scout and there was a weekend camping trip coming up. As it approached and Tom became more unwell we talked about whether Charlie still wanted to go. At first he said that he didn't, but after it became clear that Tom was slowly slipping away, he decided that he did want to go. I told him that at any time I could come and get him if he wanted me to. I remember talking to Tom about Charlie going away and we saw him give a slow blink to say to us that he thought it was OK. One of the boys' cousins would be going on the camp too, and so I thought that it would be a safe place for Charlie to be, amongst his friends and other family.

I actually breathed a sigh of relief when Charlie went off with his sleeping bag that Friday night. I knew he was scared about Tom dying and what would happen in those hours at home. Tom died the next day at 11.15 p.m., and so I decided to wait until morning to contact the scout leader to break the news. When my sister spoke to her, she said that Charlie was absolutely fine and that if it suited us, to pick him up as planned later that afternoon. It gave me some time to prepare myself for him. I am ashamed to say that I couldn't face telling Charlie myself.

One of my sisters and a close friend went to collect him and my heart just broke again as I watched him come into our living room to face me. There were no words and so he just sat on my lap and we hugged and hugged. I didn't want to let him go. He asked where Tom was and I said that he had been taken to the undertakers to rest in the chapel until the funeral could be planned. Relief, I think, washed over his face as he realized that his brother wasn't still in the house despite having died and I felt comforted that the right decisions had been made. He could remember Tom lying in bed with all his favourite things around him.

Over the course of the next two days the house was a blur of activity, with people calling in to offer their condolences. Again, I think Charlie found this difficult to witness and so he asked if he could go out for the day with one of his school friends. I think he was trying to grasp some normality and I don't blame him. The first two days after Tom died felt like we were in limbo as it was a Sunday followed by a bank holiday and so we were unable to make any plans for his funeral.

Although Charlie didn't come with me to organize the funeral, I wanted to keep him as informed as possible about what would be happening. When we went to the florists to choose the flowers, he was quite sure that he wanted sunflowers as it was always a part of our gardening rituals to plant sunflower seeds to see who could grow the tallest one. He also wanted to release a white dove at the grave, which we arranged with the undertaker.

I recall that taking Charlie shopping to buy something to wear for the funeral was quite traumatic too—although only in the respect of trying to get a nine-year-old boy to be interested in something to wear that wasn't usually a part of his wardrobe! I didn't want the funeral to be a formal affair and I was adamant that I wanted it to be 'child friendly' as I knew there would be quite a few children there. I loved that Charlie said he wanted to wear Tom's boots for it with the trousers and shirt he had chosen!

That evening we were visited by Jan, the minister who would take the service. We hadn't met before and so she sat with Charlie and me asking about Tom. Unfortunately, our cat had died the day before (I always like to think that he chose to go with Tom, who loved him!) and when Jan asked Charlie if he would perhaps like to put something in Tom's coffin, Charlie made us all laugh by saying the cat! I should add that he didn't! But he did write a letter to Tom (it was completely private and I did not read it), which I took and tucked into Tom's hand the evening before the funeral.

On the day of the funeral I could sense the concern that Charlie had for me. And I knew that Charlie would not enjoy being the focus of such attention either. He was so very brave and I was incredibly proud to have him by my side. It was so moving to watch him gently take the pure white dove from its basket and release it after the service and then be the first to drop a brightly coloured flower onto Tom's coffin. We were blessed with a fine day, and to see Charlie and his cousins playing in the garden afterwards was a huge relief although I knew that this was only the beginning of our journey through our grief.

Charlie was determined to go back to school the following week and so I arranged to go in with him later than the other children and meet with his head teacher. We were told that his class knew of his loss and were looking forward to having him back. I am grateful to his head teacher for attending the funeral as I felt it was important for Charlie to see a familiar face for him in particular.

A week after Tom's funeral we had his birthday. I knew that I would find it unbearable to be at home and so I jumped at the chance to stay with friends when invited. I think that at times like that I had to do some intuitive parenting and try to make Charlie aware that there were some things that needed to be done without question. I knew that to be with family on Tom's birthday would be extremely difficult for us and so I made the decision to take Charlie away for the weekend, where I knew he would be safe and relaxed.

Over the next few months, Charlie would often mention Tom in the context of looking down on us. Usually that he would be laughing at some misfortune that was bestowed on us, such as being stuck in traffic or getting wet in the rain. I admired this ability to hold on to Tom's character in our lives without him.

I knew that it was important for Charlie to have routine to his days, and as I mentioned in the previous chapters it was this that gave my empty days some form of structure too. As the months ticked by, I could tell that we were both being so very careful not to upset each other. There were times when having just the two of us in the house felt very intense, and rightly or wrongly I felt that I had to remain strong for Charlie, and vice versa.

When I first joined the parents' group at Helen and Douglas House, I asked Charlie if he would like some support of his own with the siblings' team but he declined. With hindsight, it feels as though we muddled along for those first couple of years.

A really important task that Charlie and I did together in that first year was to make arrangements for Tom's headstone. We visited Memorials by Artists in Suffolk to discuss what we would like to have. They specialize in bespoke headstones, in particular for children. As soon as we reached the wonderful house that served as the office and I saw Charlie wandering around the examples of headstones that were scattered amongst the most beautifully natural garden, I knew that this was what we wanted. We were put in touch with Robin Golden-Hann, the artist who would design and create the memorial. Charlie and I travelled down to Hampshire to meet him and he had thoughtfully arranged for a little carving area for Charlie to have a go at and really encouraged him to think of some ideas to incorporate into the stone. Over the next few months we then travelled to North Wales to select a piece of slate from a quarry to use as the headstone. Charlie had a wonderful time clambering up heaps of slate, looking for interesting pieces to bring home with him and also a piece that could be carved that we could keep with us at home.

Charlie decided that he would like to include Pippin, our labrador, on the headstone and so, on the back, his big tail is carved curling around the base of the stone. Encouraged by Robin we also had him carve a secret message on the part of the stone that would be hidden under ground, unknown to anybody except us. This knowledge makes me smile every time I visit the cemetery.

Just before Tom's first anniversary, Charlie and I attended a service of remembrance at Great Ormond Street Hospital. It was so very emotional to be amongst so many families who shared our loss. We sat listening to parents and siblings giving readings and poems for their loved ones, and afterwards I asked Charlie if he would like to read something out at the small service we were having on Tom's first anniversary to unveil his headstone. He agreed, and so he read out this quote by Victor Frankl that had been included in the service:

> We cannot judge a biography by its length,
>   by the number of pages in it:
>   We must judge it by the richness of the content.
>   Sometimes the 'unfinished' is among the most
>   beautiful of symphonies.

I often noticed that Charlie would refer to Tom in his school work. I will never forget seeing some of his work in history: he had been asked to write a timeline of world events and there alongside the reign of Henry VIII and the Second World War was Tom dying. Although Charlie might not say too much about losing his brother, it was obvious that is was hugely important to him. I asked him if his teacher had asked him about this inclusion, and I was a little concerned that he told me no. I have often been surprised to read in other pieces of school work snippets of life both with and without Tom that have been included.

When Charlie was twelve and at secondary school, he experienced some difficult times which were directly related to his grief. The subject of his brother was very personal and private to Charlie and not something that he felt was open for discussion for everyone. As a result of these difficult times, he was offered some support at school by Grief Encounter, a local organization for bereaved children. I found it incredibly hard not being privy to what Charlie shared with his counsellor, Yvonne, in terms of confidentiality but was relieved to hear that she found him to be a thoughtful and compassionate child in spite of the risk-taking behaviour he had taken that had resulted in him being given some support. I was naturally devastated that it had come to this, particularly when I had often offered him support in the past.

I am grateful to his school for providing the opportunity for Charlie to have this much needed input despite the circumstances in which it came about. I researched publications by the Child Bereavement Charity about a school's role in the life of a bereaved child and I passed this information on to his head of year. I think it gave Charlie the chance to realize that his grief was a very real thing but that he couldn't allow it to be a destructive force in his life. I feel that he has come out on the other side of this time with a much greater understanding of his own feelings.

One of the things that I recall discussing with his counsellor was the significance of him being the same age then as Tom was when he died. I was told that this milestone was a massive thing for Charlie and that I shouldn't have been so surprised. Although Charlie didn't give me many details of the time he spent with Yvonne, he seemed to relish the time that he did spend with her. He had a workbook which they worked on together during their sessions, and when he showed it to me I was surprised to see the words *boredom* and *bored* appearing so often. I discussed this with Yvonne and she explained to me that those were the words that Charlie used to describe his grief. They were the words he used to talk about the huge hole left in his life by the death of his brother. When asked to use colour to describe emotions and where they could be found in relation to our house, red appeared in Tom's room, and I wondered if this signified anger. Another exercise that Charlie did with Yvonne was to select a picture that he felt represented himself in a playground scene. There were illustrations depicting children and activities, and he chose the one of a child climbing up a climbing frame. I read this as him seeing his life as a bit of a struggle and it made me feel incredibly sad.

At this time Charlie also had some support from the siblings' team at Helen and Douglas House, although he declined the invitation to be involved in group sessions. As we had never stayed at the hospice as a family, I can understand his hesitation at being put into a group of children who were unfamiliar to him but with the common thread of having lost a sibling.

My thoughts on how Charlie has conducted himself over the years are that he has done so with a huge amount of maturity and dignity. For his sake, I have rarely allowed myself to fall apart in front of him and so I believe that he has mirrored this behaviour. This makes me both proud and sad at the same time as I would hate to think that he has to suppress his feelings in front of me.

I have made the decision to make sure that I am at home for the rest of Charlie's school days and I only hope that in years to come he will be able to look back and appreciate why I made that choice.

There have been times when it has been terribly difficult to allow Charlie to grow and develop; to allow him the freedom and opportunities that are all part of growing up. When he was at primary school it was a long time before I felt I could allow him to go on a school trip, because Tom had become ill as a direct result of a nursery school trip to a farm. As I became aware that he could be potentially missing out on such educational opportunities, I allowed him to go as long as I was able to attend as a helper.

During the first few weeks of him being at secondary school, a big test presented itself to me: a week-long skiing trip to the Pyrenees.

He was so keen to go, as was I to allow him to have the experience, but it felt like one of the longest weeks of my life while he was away and I was so emotional waving goodbye to him on the coach.

As Charlie grows into a teenager I am faced with many situations where all my natural instincts scream 'no', but I realize that I must allow him to do the things that his friends and peers do without hesitation. When he has pushed boundaries it has always been foremost in my mind whether the things he has done and said are because of his grief or just a normal part of adolescent behaviour. I have always stressed to him, though, that he must not use his grief as an excuse for bad behaviour per se.

I feel very aware that we have quite a unique relationship as a mother and son because our lives have shared such sadness.

Professional Perspective

What does it mean to a child or young person to have a brother or sister who dies, and how best can you support them? As with adults, the experience for your child will vary depending on the relationship they had with their sibling, whether the death was sudden or following a lengthy illness, and how much support they feel they have. It might also be influenced by how they are told of the death, and of course cultural background and religious beliefs will play a role. The biggest issue though will be what children understand about death, and that will vary according to their age and cognitive development. Understanding what death means to a child at different ages and developmental stages will give you a better idea of how to explain things to them and may also prepare you for some of their responses and questions.

A child's understanding of death develops alongside his or her cognitive maturation. Typically, below the age of five, a child does not understand that death is final and irreversible and this will come across loud and clear in the questions children of this age ask: 'When is my brother coming back?' or 'When can I see my sister again?'. While these questions are distressing for parents, they represent the child's lack of understanding that death is final. Alongside that, most pre-schoolers will not grasp that all body functions cease with death, and we know that many of them ask questions along the lines of 'Who's looking after Sam now?' or 'Who will give Ben breakfast?'. Again, these comments or questions can be painful for you as parents to hear—and they will come repeatedly—but they come from a place of good intent as they represent a child's concern for his or her sibling's well-being. It will be important in talking with your pre-schooler to use the 'D' words—death, dead, dying—and to explain that when someone dies, everything stops, so they no longer need to be fed or cared for. It is also good to explain that they no longer feel anything, so will not be cold or hungry or in pain. You might be able to draw on other experiences to help you make this clear. If you have had a family pet which has died, or have even just seen a dead bird in the garden or park, you may be able to remind your child of that and help them to understand that when a body dies it stops completely and does not come alive again.

Atle Dyregov, in his book *Grief in Children*,[1] points out that children of this age often have a circular concept of time. They experience their lives as a series of repeated loops. The daily routines, through which they move each day, repeatedly come back to the beginning and the routine begins all over again. This colours young children's understanding of death as something that is reversible. In their universe the cycle repeats itself and so they may expect that someone or something which is dead will at some point be alive again. There are also many children's stories and films where characters who have 'died' reappear, so it is not surprising that children find it hard to understand the finality of death.

While children of this age have a limited understanding of what it means to be dead, they can still react strongly to loss, often with feelings of anger or sadness. The displays of emotion may, however, be short-lived before the child is taken up with his or her normal activities. Do not be surprised if your child goes from intense crying to running off to play, in what seems like microseconds. This is not unusual behaviour in a child of this age.

Primary school age children understand death as something that cannot be changed or reversed. Put simply, they know that dead means dead, and in contrast to their younger peers recognize that all body functions come to an end. Dyregov reports that around the age of seven children come to understand that death is universal, that everyone will die and that it is unavoidable. They will also develop a more concrete understanding of the causes of death and recognize that accidents or violence may be a factor alongside illness and old age. Children in this age group are very interested in some of the more gruesome aspects of the process of dying and decomposition. As with the 'When is Sam coming back?' questions of younger children, this age group's fascination with what is happening to their brother or sister buried in the ground can be painful to hear and seem impossible to answer. It may be helpful to remind yourself that these questions are not asked to wound but are in fact genuine attempts to understand what is happening. Although these questions often come up at inopportune moments, it is good to respond with honesty whenever possible and to avoid closing down the conversation.

In adolescence the young person's concept of death will become more abstract and he or she will be able to understand some of the long-term consequences of loss. Nick, who was in his mid teens when his brother died, was acutely aware of having lost not only the day to day connectedness with his brother, but also that his brother would not be there when he graduated from college or got married. These future losses were real and significant for him. The adolescent will also be able to reflect on the fairness or unfairness of situations and the ability to think hypothetically allows him or her to ponder the 'what ifs . . .'. Amanda's bereavement support involved looking at the 'what if', relating to an earlier diagnosis of her sister's cancer and also at different treatment options. Experiencing bereavement in this age group (as with adults) may also lead to a questioning or possible rejection of previously held beliefs and values.

Whatever their children's age, parents worry about whether the child's reaction or behaviour is normal. It is not unusual for some separation anxiety to reappear, and it may mean that your child is a bit more clinging than usual. This may be more obvious in younger children, but can be true across the board. This may make transitions, for example from home to school, more difficult. Sometimes children can be helped, by taking a little bit of home with them—a favourite toy or a photograph of the family might be examples. One mum I knew gave her pre-school son a 'lipstick kiss' pressed onto a tissue, which he kept folded in his pocket, but was with him when he needed reassurance or reminding that his mum was there for him.

Sleep disturbances are also common. You may find that in the short term your child will want to sleep in your bed rather than be alone. Children might also have trouble falling asleep, as those moments without the distraction of day-to-day activities leave space for difficult thoughts. With younger children it would not be surprising to see some regression. This might mean that a child temporarily loses a skill which he or she has developed, for example you might see bed-wetting in a child who has been 'dry' or a return to other behaviours that fit a younger age.

Grief affects concentration in children as well as in adults; therefore schoolwork may become more challenging and a source of frustration. School age children and adolescents will be aware of being different from their peers and as a result may feel quite isolated. At Helen and Douglas House some of the most consistent feedback we have had from young people about our sibling support groups is that they are a place where they feel normal, rather than different. They really value being with other young people who understand, because they are going through similar things themselves. It will be infrequently that they experience that with peers.

Children are often acutely aware of their parents' pain and grief and choose to protect them from their own feelings. In combination with feeling isolated from peers this can leave some children with a real sense of loneliness and a lack of support. A support group, as I just mentioned, may make a difference. It will though be helpful for the whole family if you can take opportunities to talk about your son or daughter who has died, sharing not just memories but feelings too. Acknowledging your own feelings may give your child permission to share theirs and create opportunities for you to think together about how to manage them.

It is easy for both parents and siblings to idealize the child who has died. This can lead to your surviving child fearing that he or she will never match up and that they are less loved or loveable. Some siblings have angrily talked about feeling as if they no longer exist and that their parents would not care so much if they had been the one to die. This can have a negative impact on their ability to cope and on their current and future self-esteem. Remembering the good and the bad (or at least the naughty) about the dead child can be healthy and children of all ages will benefit from reassurance that they continue to be special and to be loved. Making equal space for each child in a family is an ongoing concern of parenthood, which does not diminish in bereavement. Try to make sure that words and behaviour match up. Your surviving child may hear that he or she is loved as much as his dead brother or sister but if the house is full of photographs of their sibling and there is little room for images of them they may not feel it rings true.

What might a child feel?

Even though a younger child may not have the words to describe what he or she is feeling, or an adolescent may simply choose not to discuss it, they do experience similar feelings to adults. This will cover the range of sadness, anger, guilt, disbelief, confusion, rage, anxiety, despair, avoidance, and longing. The feelings may be contained and not shared or they may be acted out, rather than talked out. As with adults there will be a movement between Stroebe and Schut's[2] restorative focus and loss focus (described in Chapter 1). A major difference though is the speed at which children and young people will shift from one to the other. Parents are sometimes shocked and wounded by the dramatic shift between their child's heartfelt display of sadness and the follow-on question 'Can I get on the Xbox now?'. This swift movement between emotion and continuing with life is something I have heard referred to as 'puddle jumping', in which the child can quickly switch off and carry on as normal until they are suddenly gripped by emotion again.

The idea that the movement between the two foci is healthy holds true for children as well as for adults, but you can expect your child to show a more marked shift between the two. This may make you wonder if the sadness is real. It usually is, but it is briefer than an adult often expects.

Like adults, some children will struggle to know what to do with all of these feelings, or maybe even to recognize what they are. When a child or young person feels overwhelmed by their feelings one response is to try to bury them. In younger children this might be done with some kind of distraction—kicking a football or playing with friends. Adolescents may also use distraction but may also attempt to manage feelings by numbing them using drugs or alcohol. Neither the burying nor the numbing will work, and often what results is an eruption of feelings which may seem completely out of proportion to the event precipitating it. Some children have described this as being like a volcano, which blows. One adolescent I worked with said she sometimes felt like a can of coke which just needs one more shake before it overflows, spilling over everything.

What do we know that might help children adjust to the death of a sibling and its impact on family life?

Creating time and space to help children talk about what is going on for them will make it less likely that feelings will build to bursting point. Maintaining some sense of normality will also help. You probably read that sentence and screamed at how abnormal everything is right now, but children do best when there are clear boundaries and expectations, which are applied consistently. What I mean by normality here is maintaining some of the family routines and expectations of how your children should behave. Now is not the time to allow children to do things they have not been permitted to do so far. If there is a regular bedtime stick with it as much as you can, especially if sleep is becoming an issue. If you have an agreement with your teenager about how late he or she may come home, stick with that too. Hold them to what you normally expect in terms of behaviour. You can legitimize the anger or sadness they are feeling while at the same time setting limits on how those feelings are released; therefore anger is understandable, but becoming involved in a fight at school or staying out all night is not an acceptable way to deal with it.

We know that memory work is an important part of supporting children and young people. Websites such as those of Winston's Wish and the Child Bereavement Charity have many suggestions and resources to help children and families with this, but memory boxes and books can be a good place to start. For a memory box it is good to try to include things which not only have significance but also relate to different senses. Along with photographs or a special toy, you or your son or daughter might want to include a blanket or item of clothing, which helps your child remember the special smell of the sibling who has died.

Both prior to a death, and certainly in bereavement, children need honest, direct, age-appropriate communication about what is happening. A child of five may not need details about a genetic condition, but as he or she is growing up that will become important to share. There needs to be consistency, too, in the information that is being given. Younger children, especially, may ask the same questions over and over again—it is their way of making sense of what is happening—and they need to hear the same explanation, regardless of whether it comes from you or your partner.

Use concrete terms and try to avoid euphemisms. As a culture we have an interesting vocabulary for death and dying, much of which avoids using those 'D' words. What do you think it might mean to a child to be told his brother has gone to sleep and will not wake up again or that his sister has gone on a journey and will not be coming back? For lots of children that will raise questions and anxieties about going to sleep: if I go to sleep now will I wake up again? What about other people I love—will they wake up too? Presenting death as a journey can also heighten separation anxiety. To a child's way of thinking, family members take journeys every day to school or work or the shops. How will they know which are the safe ones and which are journeys from which people may not return. I talked earlier about some children becoming a bit clingier following a death and that could be compounded by explaining it in terms of a journey. We sometimes talk with children about relatives who have died 'watching over us'. The intent of that is comforting, but again we know that this could create confusion for children with their very literal minds: 'If I'm being watched over, does that mean I have to behave all the time?'.

Children also need repeated reassurance that they are in no way responsible for what has happened. Younger children do something called 'magical thinking', in which they have some grandiose ideas about the power of their thoughts or wishes. Many parents feel that their children's wishes do have great power, but this takes it on to a whole new level! If your child has been angry or resentful of their sibling and at some point has wished that he or she would die or go away and then the child does, in fact, die, there is a strong possibility that your son or daughter will see his or her wish as causing the death. As a result your child may feel enormous guilt and responsibility for what has happened. It is incredibly important in explaining either a diagnosis of a life-limiting illness or the death of a sibling that the child is made aware that no one, least of all he or she, has caused this to happen. Do not wait until your child asks about this, because there is a strong possibility that guilt or shame would stop them from asking whether it is their fault. Make sure that in explaining what has happened to their brother or sister you include the idea that no one has made this happen.

A death impacts on a child's sense of security as it does with an adult. This, therefore, is a time when they need a constant, safe person whom they recognize is there for them. Many parents feel it a huge ask when they are engulfed by their own grief to also meet their son's or daughter's increasing needs. If it is more than you feel able to do, try to think about who else might be there for your child. Is there a grandparent or another close family member? Does your child have a teacher or activity leader who could help them?

This leads us to think about the role your child's school might play. Do let the school know what is happening, and if you can, talk with them before your son or daughter returns following the death. They may have questions for you or your child about what information is to be shared about the death and whether your child wants to be part of that or whether the teacher might explain to the other children. You might at some point want to talk with teachers about significant dates or events (birthdays, the anniversary of the death) which may be difficult times for your child. If you have any concerns, check with the school and the teachers and hear at first hand how your child is managing in the classroom. Most childhood bereavement services offer information and support to school staff responding to bereavement. If the school seems uncertain as to how to handle the situation, there are resources available to them.

Parents often have questions about the rights or wrongs of a sibling seeing their brother or sister after they have died or of attending the funeral. I think what is important is that a child is given the opportunity to be involved and is not excluded. Choice and careful preparation are the keys here. At many children's hospices families have the use of a cooled bedroom, where the child who has died is cared for between the time of death and the funeral. Siblings may be given the option of spending some time there and if they choose to do this they should have some idea of what to expect: a description of the room— at Helen and Douglas House, for example, it is just another bedroom—and what their sibling will look and feel like will help them perhaps with the decision of whether to go in or not, and if they do it will give them some idea of what it might be like. Some advance warning of how cold the bedroom is will help too. In my experience the majority of siblings, from pre-schoolers up, have chosen to go or followed their parents in to see their brother or sister and have also decided when they no longer felt the need or desire to spend any more time there. They have been involved with decorating the room with drawings or photographs and perhaps choosing a toy or writing a letter to put in the coffin.

Similar choice and preparation need to be given about attending or participating in the funeral. Current thinking is that it is beneficial for children to be involved, but again I think it is important to encourage children to take part in farewell rituals but to respect choice. An explanation about what will happen and that the funeral is about saying goodbye to their brother or sister may help a child decide if they want to participate or not. If they choose to come, you may like to ask someone your child knows and trusts if they would be available to look after them during the service, including taking them out if needed. Surviving siblings can often make great contributions when planning a service as they may know inside out what their brother or sister would have enjoyed or appreciated and, equally, what they would not have liked. Sometimes siblings will want to take part in the service, perhaps by writing something or performing a piece of music or song. It can be a good idea to have a back-up plan as sometimes a child may be overwhelmed by the moment and find it harder to stand up and do something than everyone is anticipating. I remember one funeral when a sibling, Chloe, with the help of our music therapist, prepared a song to sing. In the days leading up to the funeral they recorded it, so that if at the funeral Chloe felt she could not go ahead with it, her tribute to her brother would still be heard.

Sometimes families choose not to include younger children because they think they will not understand what is happening and will not remember it in later life. Dyregov[1] talks, though, about how some of these young children as they grow up are glad to have been involved in such a significant family event. They may not remember it, but it means a lot to them that they were included.

As with adults, a child's grief will change over time, but for children the changes will not just be in how they feel but also in what their grief means at different points in their life. We know that children will do some reworking of their grief as they mature and develop a different understanding of the meaning of death. There will also be significant transitional points for them, for example younger siblings growing to be older than their deceased brother or sister or developing skills which their sibling did not survive to achieve. This could include moving from junior to senior school, a first job, or going away to university. Achievements like making it onto the football team or learning to drive could also trigger some resurgent sadness. As parents, these same events may also have an impact on you. Be aware that they may resonate with your child too and that he or she may need more support at these points, or at least the chance to talk about what is happening.

Just as you may struggle with questions about how many children you have, siblings can be troubled by the idea of their position in the family being realigned. They need time to question or process the idea of now being an 'only child' or moving from being a younger sibling to perhaps being the older sibling. Like you, they too will keenly feel the impact of the changed composition of the family and will also need time to come to terms with it. A twelve-year-old girl whose family I supported spoke very articulately about not wanting to turn sixteen as this would technically make her older than her big brother, who had died shortly before his sixteenth birthday. In the first year after her brother died she did not look forward to school holidays the way she had before. It was not just that Joseph was no longer there, but neither were the carers and all the activity that surrounded them. She was very aware of the relative emptiness of the house and of the changing dynamics of a family of three as opposed to a family of four plus. We will talk about planning for significant dates, holidays etc in a later chapter, but what is important to stress here is the value of talking these changes through with children.

In closing this chapter I want to share something from one of our sibling support groups as I think it sums up some of what this experience is like for children. At the end of a morning session of a very gradual and gentle introduction to acting out different emotions and states, the children were asked to put together a two-minute performance for which the topic was 'I wish...'. They came up with their individual 'I wish' and then worked in pairs before doing their presentation in a group of four. When it came to the presentations every single group of four acted out a variation of a very typical and age-appropriate wish, for example 'I wish my house was made of sweets', alongside the more poignant 'I wish my brother or sister was still alive'. They may be sad and grieving, but they are also children and we will serve them best by recognizing that and allowing them to be who and what they are.

Things to Remember

What I have written about in this chapter relates to children in general. How your son or daughter reacts to grief will of course be a very personal experience. Your knowledge of your own child will be key to trying to work out how best to support them. Here though are some pointers to what bereaved children might benefit from:

- Honest, age-appropriate information, which may need to be repeated
- Recognition of their feelings
- Permission and encouragement to talk about their sibling
- Reassurance that they are in no way to blame
- Consistency and continuity
- Opportunities to create and/or retain memories
- Time just to be a child

References

1. Dyregov, A. (2008) *Grief in children: a handbook for adults*, 2nd revised edn. Jessica Kingsley Publishers, London.
2. Stroebe, M. and Schut, H. (1999) The dual process model of coping with bereavement: rationale and description. *Death Studies*, **23**, 197–224.

Your Notes

Chapter 4

The impact of grief on couples

Parent's Perspective

I am very aware that so far in this book I have made no mention of a husband or partner; the simple reason for this is that when Tom died I had been divorced from John, the boys' father, for some years. On reflection I could say that it was grief that was a major factor in us separating; we separated within a year of Tom becoming ill and so we were, in fact, grieving for the loss of the child who we had known.

When Tom was transferred back to our local hospital in August 1997, his father went back to work. I felt abandoned and angry that his work could become the priority for him, as I had no regard for practicalities such as paying the mortgage and bills. My sole focus was on my children. I simply didn't understand how such a decision could be made. I have talked to many bereaved mothers and they have voiced similar feelings of abandonment when their husband or partner has returned to work. As the full impact of being responsible for creating a new kind of life for me and my children became apparent I was forcibly made to reconsider my priorities in life, and it seemed that the lowest priority I had was being a wife. I knew that I had a huge amount of learning to do, and I eventually made the decision that I didn't want a passenger on this journey. It seemed very heartless, but I felt desperate that the energy I had should go into the survival of my children and not into putting right the tatters that my marriage was in. There was a massive lack of communication, and not only was I unable to express how I felt but I was also disappointed and hurt in that I didn't feel as if I was getting any emotional support. I simply did not have the strength to support another person.

Over the following nine years, the relationship I had with my ex-husband became distant and less important to me, other than in trying to allow some form of contact with the boys. As time passed, he found himself in a new relationship and so it was as if his life had moved on and mine had remained the same. Don't get me wrong—I felt no bitterness or sadness, because it had been my decision to part and so he was free to do whatever he felt was right.

As Tom's prognosis became more apparent I had to share this with his father, and because he was so uninvolved in our day-to-day life it was a huge burden for me to have to break this news to him. Again, I was lucky to have an extremely supportive team and I arranged for a meeting to be held at the hospital for us to attend together for the news to be broken to him. I remember feeling guilty and embarrassed that such decisions had even been talked about without him present, but equally that he hadn't been there at crucial moments to witness why these decisions had been made.

During Tom's last few days at home, his father was at our house for some of the time—taking care of Charlie and getting the shopping. The burden of being Tom's main carer seemed overwhelming, and I felt as though I had to prove myself in being competent in what I was doing as it was my choice to have Tom at home. When Tom died, his dad had to be brought from Charlie's bedroom as he had gone to bed. This was the most alien thing to me as it felt as though wild horses wouldn't have dragged me away from my child. It was one of many, many times when I realized that men and women are inexplicably different. Likewise, I recall hearing him making conversation with the undertakers outside the house at 4 a.m. when they had come to take Tom. I couldn't even have looked at them, let alone talked to them, even out of politeness.

It has often been commented to me that it is dreadful that I had to experience losing my child on my own, but I have never really dwelt on it, mostly I think because I have always been very aware that it was my decision. I do know that I felt lonelier in my marriage than I did when I left it to be on my own.

When Tom had first become ill it was as though a self-protection mechanism kicked in and the thing that was sacrificed was my own ability to maintain an intimate relationship with anyone. After Tom died, I felt that an impenetrable steel cage had surrounded me—I felt that I couldn't cope with people seeing the extent of my grief, but I didn't know how to acknowledge the grief they were feeling too. I could barely look myself in the eye, let alone look at anybody else. I would liken it to a learnt behaviour in my coping skills: when there didn't seem to be anyone to support me emotionally, I learnt to do without.

When I first started attending workshops at Helen and Douglas House, I found it excruciatingly difficult to watch couples expressing their grief, not only to each other but also to the rest of the room. I had never before witnessed such genuine grief from any man. It upset me enormously and I realized that none of us would ever have exactly the same experience.

With hindsight, I actually consider myself lucky that I was able to concentrate on my needs and those of Charlie without having to support another person. I often felt comfortably selfish in only having to consider what was right for me. I felt that the way I was behaving was very instinctive, and knowing what sort of person I am I would have felt very challenged if there was somebody present who potentially could have criticized the way I was doing things. I felt that it was my right after everything I had gone through to do exactly as I pleased. Having said that, I constantly questioned myself and spent many hours discussing the way I felt with Christine and the other parents in my group. It was only when I was in the company of other bereaved parents that I allowed myself to accept that how I felt, in spite of being a single parent, was acceptable and, dare I say it, normal.

The thread of the difficulties faced when a spouse returns to work after losing a child is one I have encountered in virtually all the contact I have had with other bereaved parents, and having already experienced it once, as I have described earlier, I have to admit to being thankful I was spared this issue for a second time around. By all accounts, it seems to be one of the biggest hurdles that couples have to face.

When it came to planning Tom's funeral, I was very aware that it shouldn't be all my decision as to how we went ahead, and so I always tried to include his dad in the procedure although it was still very much left to me to make the choices. Maybe too much time had passed for him to feel that his opinion was needed. I felt very conspicuous standing on one side of the chapel while he stood on the other, with his partner and family, but at the same time something very strong within me made me feel that putting on a united front for the sake of the congregation was wrong. I had always felt I had been true to Tom and now that feeling remained in that I had to remain true to myself. In my darker moments I often wondered if Charlie had felt torn being between his parents on such an occasion.

The relationship I now have with the boys' dad remains as distant as it has always been since we separated, and we both lead our own very private lives, with the one connection now being Charlie. We do not mark any special occasions together, such as Tom's birthday or anniversary, and this is a mutual, if unsaid, agreement.

Professional Perspective

Not long after I began working at Helen and Douglas House I was supporting a family whose toddler son had died two days previously. Their little boy, Andrew, was in the cooled bedroom and his parents were staying in one of the family flats. I clearly remember going into the flat and finding them distressed by a book they had found, which suggested that more than seventy per cent of bereaved parents ultimately divorce. I was struck by the added worry this created for them. They were only beginning to contemplate a life without their much-loved son and now were also anxious that they might lose each other. Up until that point they had experienced the normal ups and downs of a committed relationship, but their reading left them asking whether the death of a child and the divorce of his parents were cause and effect.

Let's clear up that myth right at the start of this discussion. High divorce rates among bereaved parents have been exaggerated. In 2006 The Compassionate Friends carried out a study of 400 bereaved parents,[1] in which they were asked about their marital status at the time of their child's death and their current marital status. This yielded a divorce rate of 16%, which confirmed the findings of an earlier study that The Compassionate Friends had conducted in the late 1990s. Of the people who had divorced, fewer than half (40%) felt that the child's death had contributed to the divorce. A paper published in 1998, entitled 'A child's death and divorce: dispelling the myth',[2] adds weight to this. The author, Reiko Schwab, examined the evidence for the higher divorce rates and found that it did not stand up. Schwab suggested that one of the factors contributing to this myth was that there was a confusion between marital distress and divorce. This makes sense, as I think that what is important to know about parental bereavement and its impact on a couple is that while the risk of divorce is relatively low, there is no question that losing a child has the potential to significantly strain a relationship. But how could it not?

In the best of circumstances, when any one of us goes through something painful and life changing our partner is typically the person we would expect to help us through it. When your child dies, that person is reeling from the same body blow that you are. It will take each of you all of your resources to get up and get through the day, and there may not be much left over to help each other. Many couples who have cared for their son or daughter for years find that they have become co-parents, rather than partners. It is hard to find the time or energy for each other when you are sleep deprived, and harder still to have time and space when care staff and other professionals frequently fill the house. That could mean that you are grieving alongside some-one who has become a relative stranger. Your child's death may mean having to rebuild that relationship. There could be a sense of finding again something which has been lost. Equally, there could be the real-ization of now having to deal with difficulties and differences which were previously swept under the carpet.

Couples who have been strong and connected before the death may feel a distance developing as each is absorbed by their own grief. If your relationship was wobbly before your child died you will have to manage the pre-existing problems in addition to the grief. A therapist colleague likens her clients' relationships to a boat. If your boat is in pretty good shape before you hit the stormy seas you will have to work hard bailing out water, but the likelihood is that you will make it through. Conversely if you are in a leaky boat to start with you will have a much bigger job to do to stop yourselves from going under. The vast majority of couples I have seen do somehow manage to stay afloat, so how do they do it? It seems to take hard work, commitment, and a degree of acceptance of each other's coping styles, but it is do-able.

What I have seen with many couples is that partners are confused or upset by how the other person is grieving. If you are someone who makes sense of things by talking and going over things and your part-ner cannot bear those kinds of conversations but perhaps spends a lot of time being busy, how do you manage that? Similarly if you are a 'doer' and your partner struggles to get out of bed and start going how do you live with that?

The essential thing is to try to set aside what your expectations are of how someone *should* grieve. In Chapter 1 I mentioned that one of the most frequent questions parents ask is 'Is this normal?' and that, in most cases, it is. The range of normal is broad, however. Many of us fall into the trap of thinking that our way of doing something or how we experience it is the right or only way. This leads us to expect that everyone else should behave similarly. A couple I worked with had very different needs in relation to how much time they spent at their daughter's grave. For the mum daily visits were part of her routine. She interpreted her husband's much less frequent visits to the grave as somehow not right (i.e. he was not grieving properly) and this created resentment and conflict between them. If you expect your partner to grieve in the same way as you do but they are doing it completely differently you are setting yourself up for disappointment. We talked earlier in this book about there being no right or wrong way to grieve. People process both experiences and emotions in a variety of ways and over differing time-scales. If your partner is behaving differently from you try not to judge him or her, and certainly do not assume that he or she finds this any less painful than you do. The likelihood is that it is equally painful but that it is being managed in a different way. Remind yourself of other experiences you have had as a couple—the birth of your child or perhaps the diagnosis of their condition. Did each of you respond to that in the same way? Most likely the answer to that question is no. Why then expect that you will grieve in the same way or for the same time? You are both parents of your child, but you each have a separate relationship with him or her which will colour what the loss means for you.

I have often been asked if there are differences in how men and women grieve. In fact this was often a discussion topic in workshops and in our bereavement support groups. I think, though, that there is no definitive answer. It has been suggested that Stroebe and Schut's dual process model[3] which we looked at earlier in the book goes some way to explaining gender differences in grief, but it is never simple when we generalize behaviours. If we remind ourselves briefly of that model, the loss-oriented focus deals primarily with the emotions of loss and the restoration focus more with tasks, distraction from grief, and new roles. An idea put forward about this model is that since women are more likely to respond to problems by talking about them and emoting they are therefore more likely to display loss-oriented behaviour. Men, who in our culture tend to want to fix problems and therefore be solution focused, are more likely to show restoration-oriented behaviour. Following a bereavement in a family known to me the response of one man was to set about painting the kitchen walls. This man's partner was aghast, but the painting was about preparing the house for the many people who would be invited there after the funeral. This man did not want to talk about what he was feeling, but was focused on the practical and what he saw as needing to be done. Of course healthy grief moves backwards and forwards between loss and restoration, and in my experience at Helen and Douglas House we see some of each of these behaviours in both men and women.

However, I do think that gender roles and expectations play a part in how men and women grieve, or at least how they show their grief. We live in a culture and society in which it is generally more acceptable for women to display emotions than it is for men. I have come across a lot of fathers who feel that they have to be strong and that strength is interpreted to mean not crying or showing any emotion, or if they do that it has to be done privately. I think a good example of that is a dad I worked with who talked about his car journey to and from work as his time and space to grieve for his daughter. In the solitude, if not complete privacy, of his car he could simply think or cry. He looked forward to his journey time to be able to do this. We talked about it in a joint support session with his wife, but without this conversation she may well have wondered about his lack of emotion or assumed that he did not feel the loss as deeply as she did. He, though, had found the time to reflect and to feel and to do it in a way that felt right for him, which was to do it privately.

Although gender roles and career paths have changed over the years, many fathers still see themselves as the family provider. And the reality for many families who have lived long term with a life-limited child is that the dad is the sole earner. This can create pressure to get back to work as soon as possible. From the outside that could be interpreted as the behaviour of someone who is not so deeply affected by the loss, but I know of many situations where dads, and sometimes mums, saw themselves as having no choice. That is especially true when someone is self-employed. In that situation not working means no income, which is not an option, especially when as well as the normal living expenses families may also be losing allowances or a mobility car and in addition have funeral expenses. I think another driver pushing dads back to work is the notion of the father not only as provider but also as protector. Whether consciously or unconsciously, a parent can interpret their child's death as a failure on their part to protect them. Ensuring that they provide financially for the remaining family is one way of containing the ensuing anxiety and is a very tangible expression of taking control and fulfilling that protective role. For the parent who has to return to work it can be an almighty struggle to get there, switch off from the raw pain, and focus on the task in hand. I have seen many situations where the parent back at work envied their partner what they saw as the luxury of being able to stay at home and take the time to think and grieve. The reality is that each role is hard. Work can be a distraction, but it may take unimaginable energy to arrive there and then survive the day. Staying at home is no picnic either. The parent at home can feel that their partner is moving on and that they are being left behind. The mere fact of the working parent being connected to the other world of work can heighten differences when the primary carer may be very isolated and even begin to view work as being pointless after the death of their child. Some parents experience their partner's return to work as another abandonment, at a time when they are especially needy. Most parents who delay their return to work, or who have no job to return to, are challenged to create a whole new structure to their day and sometimes a whole new identity, which we looked at in Chapter 2.

The bottom line is that grieving is hard work for each of you, and cultural, role, and personality differences will influence how each of you navigates it. Try not to interpret your partner's behaviour, or make assumptions about what it means, especially not using your own coping style as the yardstick by which you measure it.

Try to talk with your partner about your feelings and about theirs, but respect when one or other of you will not or cannot have that conversation.

In Chapter 1 we talked a little about grief and its impact on sexuality. For some couples this aspect of their relationship continues as before, while for others it can become either a pressure or another potential loss. If you had a healthy sex life while your son or daughter was alive hopefully that will continue. Some couples find that sex or their attitude to it changes with grief. One partner may feel guilt at doing anything pleasurable, including sex, which can lead to the avoidance of intimacy or having sex and feeling bad about it afterwards. Someone else may find that grief increases the need for closeness and that sometimes sex can provide that. If you are at different points on this spectrum your needs will be mismatched. Also if you are someone for whom emotional intimacy is a requirement for physical intimacy, and grief is creating distance between you and your partner, there is a potential problem. If sex really becomes an issue between you, you may for a time at least want to think about finding other ways to remain intimate and connected with each other.

What can couples do about these challenges? As with almost every other relationship issue the single most important strategy is to keep the communication going between you. Explaining to your partner either that you cannot face sex or that you desperately want to be close will help him or her understand what is happening and make it less likely that he or she will feel either rejected or pressured. The danger in not talking, whether about feelings or sexuality, is that misunderstandings grow and they will fuel arguments and distance. The greater the distancing, the harder it will be to bridge the gap between you.

When you are in the middle of something as painful as grief it is hard to think forward to a time when things might feel less tortuous, but remind yourself that however you feel at this particular moment it will change. It is all too easy to allow this particular snapshot of your relationship to grow and to project it into the future. It does not have to happen that way. Feeling misunderstood by your partner or struggling with their need for or lack of interest in sex does not have to be a continuous state. Remember that by far the majority of couples survive this.

Real life does not stop while you are grieving, so you will still have to negotiate the normal day-to-day issues that are the fodder of many arguments. If you have surviving children they will also have needs, which may increase following the death of their sibling. They need a sense of safety and security, so it is good to maintain the regular boundaries and for you and your partner to be consistent with this. When one or both of you is drained it is tempting to slacken the rules, but try to think through the consequences. Trade off the parental roles that perhaps feel too much for either of you and allow other people to help too.

Again the key is to talk things through, check things out, and negotiate. That will be particularly important not just with the day-to-day responsibilities but also with significant dates and events. Birthdays and anniversaries of all kinds will take on a different meaning now. You may want to maintain your usual traditions, but for some you will have to create new ones. Again try not to make any assumptions about what each of you will or will not want to do. Talk about each one as it approaches and respect that you may not always want to handle it the same way. One father felt strongly that on the first anniversary he wanted to take off for open space and the coast, whereas the mother was determined to remain where her child had died for that anniversary.

There is a degree to which everyone finds ways of deadening the pain. For some parents it can be physical activity or fundraising, for others it might be spending time with people who knew and loved your child. Some parents find that alcohol brings a temporary release. It may briefly take the edge off the pain or it may permit tightly held emotions to be released. That may have an occasional benefit, but if it becomes habitual or escalates it will be counter-productive. A hangover will make the days harder to get through—you will have even less energy and your mood will be further depressed. It may also contribute to or escalate conflict in the family. Again if you see this becoming a problem you have to address it with your partner and perhaps seek professional support.

If, as in Tracy's case, you have previously separated from your child's father or mother you may find the loss of your child reopening some of the painful emotions of your relationship. It is also likely that at the time of death and for a little while afterwards you will be required to have increased contact. Trying to sort out funeral arrangements or your child's belongings with a former partner may require more energy and support than if you were still together. Given that extended family members may also have some negative emotions for this person, you might find yourself in an emotional minefield. At Helen and Douglas House we have worked with families to help them have these conversations. Having someone who is not emotionally involved help each of you hear what the other is saying may allow you to stay focused on the task in hand.

Apart from keeping the communication open, what else can help? Even at the best of times no one person can meet all of another person's needs. Think about who else you have in your life who can share in supporting you. If your partner cannot tolerate another discussion about your child's final hours or the medical decisions you made and you have a need to go over it time after time, is there a friend or family member who can listen? Can you allow neighbours or co-workers to provide the meals they are offering so that you have a little more energy for your relationship? Is there a bereavement support group you can join, either individually or as a couple? A group would give you time and space to share your grief with people who can hear and understand it. You would also get to see and hear how others are coping and that might give you some new ideas or help you understand your own or your partner's perspective. In seeing how other parents react you might even recognize that your partner is not being so unusual or difficult after all! A small example of this is a discussion at one of the Helen and Douglas House parent support groups in which parents discovered that, in most couples, one of them had read everything they could find about grief and was irritated and confused by their partner's lack of interest. The shared discussion assisted the parents to try to see it from another point of view and to begin to recognize that maybe what was important for them was not so for everyone. I also know that for some parents it was by coming to our groups and workshops that they found out what was going on with their partner. In the safety of the group they were able to share things which perhaps seemed too risky or potentially uncontainable to talk about at home.

Most hospices for children and young adults offer bereavement support to parents either individually or as a couple. If this is available to you, you may want to try it. An experienced bereavement worker should be able to help you make sense of your grieving and hopefully help you to hear each other. If your difficulties are less grief related then you might want to think about a relationship counsellor. Although the majority of bereaved parents do stay together, there will be couples who decide to separate, and doing this with the help of a professional will allow you to talk about what needs to happen without tearing each other apart.

In conclusion, let's remind ourselves of where this chapter began. High divorce rates among bereaved parents have been exaggerated. Most relationships survive the death of a child. Most probably you and your partner will grieve differently and that may strain your relationship, but it does not have to break it. And at the risk of being really repetitive, a large part of the solution lies in communicating.

Things to Remember

- Divorce rates among bereaved parents have been exaggerated
- Expect to grieve differently from your partner
- Try not to make assumptions about your partner's behaviour
- No one person can meet your needs, so think about who else can be there for you
- Communication is key

References

1. The Compassionate Friends (2006) *When a child dies* [a survey of bereaved parents]. Available at: http://www.compassionatefriends.org/pdf/When_a_Child_Dies-2006_Final.pdf
2. Schwab, R. (1998) A child's death and divorce: dispelling the myth. *Death Studies*, **22**, 445–68.
3. Stroebe, M. and Schut, H. (1999) The dual process model of coping with bereavement: rationale and description. *Death Studies*, **23**, 197–224.

Your Notes

Chapter 5

Grandparents, extended family, and friends

Parent's Perspective

When Tom died, one of the things I will always remember is my dad just saying 'I'm your dad'. At the time it struck me as a really peculiar thing to say but as years have passed I have begun to realize the significance of his statement: it was as though it was the only thing he could say to me.

The relationship with my parents since then has been very much up and down. In the early days, if I were to be brutally honest, I felt totally abandoned by everybody. It felt as though everyone was completely caught up in their own grief (which, of course, they were) and were leaving me and Charlie to ours. I recall feeling extremely angry that my sister, for example, had what I considered to be a long time off work afterwards. I felt that I didn't have the luxury of having time off from anything to adjust to my changed life.

I had such a conflict of emotions running through me—although I felt as lonely as I'd ever felt in my entire life, when people did try to reach out to me I didn't feel able to talk to them. My phone would ring, and I would just let it ring out. If I did answer, I would be monosyllabic and untalkative, often resorting to the stock answer of 'I'm fine' to enquiries as to how I was doing.

In family situations, I felt so uncomfortable because it was as though my family had been torn apart, never to be the same again. It was as if there was a gaping hole.

The thing was, I didn't know what I needed from anyone. I was very aware that my parents and other close family had their own grief and I unconsciously made the decision that I was unable to support them and so it was as though I cut myself off from them. In essence, I really didn't know what I wanted or needed. All I knew was that I was doing everything I could to get through my days. I felt very protective and defensive about my grief. It made me feel even more disappointed when I discovered that my family would ask my friends how I was but never ask me. It highlighted the communication void that existed between us all. I remember in the lead up to the first Christmas without Tom, my mum asked if I would be coming out on an annual girls' Christmas dinner. When I replied that I wouldn't be this year, I was astonished when she asked me why not. What bit didn't she understand?

Another thing I was acutely aware of was that, fourteen years earlier, my youngest sister had lost twin boys as babies, and after I had lost Tom our other sister must have had thoughts of whether she would be next in line. We never actually discussed this, but I was always very conscious that she may feel dreadfully uncomfortable.

I was so angry in those first few months of losing Tom, and I can recognize that I directed much of the anger into the way I felt about my family. It was as though they were the closest targets. It's not that I ranted and raved at them, it was more of a slow simmering just below the surface. I would get really frustrated at the fact that my parents made a weekly trip to the cemetery to put flowers on Tom's grave. It made me angry that they could go there but ignore the fact that they had another grandchild who was still alive but not worthy of their time.

Once I started attending workshops and my parents group at Helen and Douglas House, I was almost relieved to hear that other parents were experiencing exactly the same kind of emotional conflicts with their families as I was. It was incredibly valuable to be able to talk openly about the way we were all feeling without being judged or contradicted.

I also found the advice of my homeopath crucial to getting me past these destructive thoughts. It was with her gentle guidance that I began to learn to accept the new me and the ways in which others are different.

I remember spending an awful lot of time in my one-to-one counselling sessions with Christine going over and over the way I felt I was dealing (or sometimes not dealing) with the way I felt about my family and friends. A huge part of coming to terms with the new me and my new life was to learn to live it differently, with perhaps a different set of values and beliefs. I had to learn that I could not be everything to everybody, no matter what I felt was expected of me. When the subject arose of whether my parents would be interested in attending a workshop at Helen and Douglas House for bereaved grandparents, I knew that there was no way they would attend unless I took them there. For that reason I didn't tell them about it, because I felt that if I had to be proactive about managing my own grief then so should they. To make up for the lack of empathy I felt from them, I went out and found other sources of support.

Within the wider circle of my family there was a huge difference in the way grief was communicated. I believe that in spite of being a geographically close family, we are not necessarily emotionally close and therefore there wasn't really ever any open talk of how much we were all grieving. From where I was, it almost felt as though everything was carrying on as before. At the time, I looked after my young nephews and niece and the innocence of their age was almost refreshing. The younger ones always wanted to talk about Tom and ask things about him and I relished the opportunity to talk together. I also noticed that they were almost blatant in the way they watched me going about things.

Over the years that followed I had the opportunity to talk about the way I felt about my family and to resolve the way I felt about them and they way they handled both my grief and their own. I learnt to accept that I couldn't change the way they did things and that I didn't have to change the way I did things to please them. Importantly, I also learnt that the anger I felt was a very common feeling in the early stages of my grief and this helped me put it into perspective as I was desperately unhappy with the way I was feeling; it felt completely irrational.

One of the other overwhelming feelings I experienced was that I had been given the chance to weed out the things or people in my life that were not important. That sounds drastic and unforgiving, but at the time I knew that my energy was low and I would need to prioritize the little I did have. I had a very small core group of friends who kept their eye on me, but even then it was often too much to talk to them. I know that there were times when they talked amongst themselves about how concerned they were to hear that each time they called to ask as to what I was doing, my reply was often that I was just sitting on the sofa. I have talked about the physical tiredness of grief in earlier chapters, but nobody really had any idea of the enormousness of feeling this way and how long it would last.

Over the course of the first two years after Tom died, I began to find other ways to communicate and make other friends and connections. I became proficient at using my computer and accessing the internet for all manner of things. I began to read the blogs of people who had similar interests to me and slowly I entered a virtual world where I could be myself (or what I considered to be a new version of myself). It was refreshing to 'meet' people who did not know my history and accept me for who I was. After a while, I started writing my own blog and as my confidence grew I felt it became necessary for me to show all my cards and so I wrote on my blog about Tom. It was one of the hardest posts I have ever written. I was amazed at the amount of support and kind words that I received from people around the world who had never met me (or Tom). They gave me the courage to write about how I felt, although I was always very careful about what I wrote. The aim of my blog was a place to notice the beauty of this world and record it and I didn't want it to have a depressing, pessimistic theme to it. My blog also gave me a space to remember Tom and acknowledge my grief. It seems somewhat of a contradiction to consider myself a very private person when I was writing about my life and publishing it on the internet, but the blogging world is a very friendly place and was exactly what I needed at the time. In fact, I still do. As Christine once said to me, that when something is missing in your life, fate often delivers an alternative even though you are not really looking for one.

Not long after I started blogging, I was given a link to an Australian blogger who was also a bereaved parent. She shared my love of crafting and so I came to believe that I could be a bereaved parent and something else too. Through blogging I found a sense of community that was lacking in my existing relationships with my family and friends. This was a revelation and the start of a new beginning for me: one where I could manage my grief, my anger, my family, and still find the inspiration to learn to live with my loss.

Professional Perspective

This far we have focused on the process of grief itself, its broader impact on the life of a family, and specifically what it means for siblings and for the parental relationship. But families extend beyond those relationships, therefore grandparents and other close family members (aunts, uncles, godparents) will be affected too.

As a grieving grandparent you can expect to go through all of the physical and emotional pain of mourning that we described in Chapter 1. Grief may have an impact on every aspect of your life, affecting how you feel physically, emotionally, and spiritually. You may feel extreme sadness or anger and in the next moment find yourself able to engage with life, taking care of daily chores or perhaps offering practical help to your bereaved son or daughter. What you will carry in addition to your own grief, however, is the added injury of watching your own son or daughter suffer and feeling powerless to do anything about it. And that in a nutshell is the dilemma for grandparents—how to manage your own grief while trying to support your adult child through something that no amount of paternal or maternal love can fix for them. Other family members and friends will also have the dual challenge of coping with their own grief and watching someone they care for suffering.

Your grief will of course be determined by your relationship with your grandchild. Many grandparents are very 'hands on' and you may have been closely involved in caring for your grandchild or in helping his or her parents. You will miss that regular contact and feel the loss intensely. Geography, other responsibilities, or a conflicted relationship may mean that you were not involved as much as you might have liked to be, in which case a sense of missed opportunity may be part of your grief. For all grandparents and extended family there is sadness at the loss of hopes for the relationship which might have developed as well as for the person who you assumed you would watch growing up. There is almost always some survival guilt too.

The death of a child is particularly shocking in that it upsets the natural order of life. Parents in our culture are not expected to outlive their children, and grandparents can feel that even more strongly. You are not the first grandparent to have thought or even voiced, 'It should have been me'. Making sense of a world in which a young life has ended when an older person continues to be alive can leave you questioning your values and beliefs. It also may leave you with survivor guilt—a sense that you should not be alive when others have died. There is no easy solution to this or to the questions which might be running around in your head, but it may help to know that other grandparents have experienced something similar. It may also help simply to acknowledge the confusion of feelings, whatever they are. However, to some of you that may seem self-indulgent.

At Helen and Douglas House we have run occasional workshops for grandparents, and with each of them the challenge for staff facilitating the sessions has been to get participants to talk about their *own* grief. Their focus has typically been not on themselves but on how they can help their adult children, the bereaved parents. That demonstrates wonderful and much needed support for their children, but they may need some of that support too. Most parents are adept at taking care of their children's needs ahead of their own, but in this instance you will possibly support your son or daughter best by acknowledging your own feelings and being supported too.

Many years ago I co-facilitated a support group with someone who used the in-flight demonstration of safety equipment as an analogy for self-care, and I think it may help illustrate the point here. One of the instructions that flight attendants give (or at least used to give) is that if during the flight the cabin pressure changes and oxygen masks are required you should put your own mask on first, before attempting to help a child or someone unable to attach the mask for themselves. It follows that you will be much better placed to be of use to your grieving son or daughter if you have the equivalent of your own oxygen mask in place, whether that is a friend with whom you can talk or someone to look after your own home while you cook or clean or just be there for the bereaved parents.

Having said that it is important to acknowledge your grief and not to struggle alone with it; a balance needs to be achieved. Many grandparents and extended family members get it right, but in my experience one of the greatest frustrations for grieving parents is any hint that this becomes about you, the grandparent, and your grief, rather than the parents' grief. In our support groups we always discourage parents from comparing grief. I remember one father suggesting that his loss was less awful than another couple's because he had surviving children and the other couple did not. There is simply no scale to measure one parent's loss against another, and neither should there be. Most grandparents are acutely aware that no matter how painful the loss is for them, it is immeasurably more difficult for their son or daughter. Sometimes, however, they or other family members do need reminding of this. There may be competing needs within a grieving family, but there should be no competition about whose pain is greater or who is more entitled to be grieving.

In many families there is an expectation that in a crisis everyone pulls together or that it will bring out the best in people. This does sometimes happen, and families do a fantastic job of supporting each other, rising to the occasion and working as a united team. Realistically, though, few of us perform at our best when we are feeling vulnerable or under enormous stress, and many of us revert to childhood family roles, which can lead to some pretty challenging behaviour. Furthermore, a child's death is not something that many people have experience of handling, so each of you may feel overwhelmed and out of your depth. If there were tensions in the family before the child died these may be magnified afterwards. This means that in addition to the pain of seeing your adult child, sibling, or friend suffer you may also be on the receiving end of some horribly difficult behaviour or conversations. Families, generally, are where we feel safe. That can mean that we save the worst of our behaviour for them. If bereaved parents have struggled to hold it together at the school gates or on returning to work, family or close friends might be the very people with whom they cannot or maybe will not hold back their emotions. You, therefore, may be the person to see the tears and receive the fury that others are shielded from. The best you can do is to simply be there. Sit with the tears, acknowledge the anger, and resist the temptation to try to fix them. There is no parental kiss or Band-Aid that will take this pain away.

What else can you do? If there are surviving children maybe you can be there for them. They too will be grieving and adjusting to the changed family composition. It is likely too that their mum or dad will not have their usual patience or energy to support them. There may also be practical things, like shopping or fielding calls, which you can take on. For any family member trying to help, the best advice is always to check first about what will be useful. Do not make any assumptions about what the bereaved family might need or want from you, but be specific about what you are offering. General offers of 'Let me know if I can do anything', are seldom taken up. A specific offer of, for example, preparing the house for people after a funeral, or of doing the garden, is something to which it is easier to respond.

While you may be trying to be there for your son, daughter, or sibling, they may choose not to share their distress with you. If they are talking to a friend or other family member or decide to get some outside help, perhaps from a bereavement counsellor, try not to feel rejected or inadequate. It may be easier for them to talk with someone who is not involved emotionally and they may also wish to protect you and other people whom they care about from some of what they are experiencing, just as you may also choose to protect them from your own pain.

Try to be sensitive about family events and occasions. It is hard to predict what will feel difficult and what will feel acceptable to be part of. Recognize that, both for yourself and also for your son or daughter. Try not to work on assumptions or guesses. Check how the bereaved parents want to handle birthdays or anniversaries and try to respect their choices. Remember, too, that significant events and transitions for other family members will take on a different meaning now. One mum I supported, Lynn, was beginning to feel life becoming a little more stable, until the birth of her nephew. Her mother had sensitively driven her to see the new baby and agreed to stay for as long or as short a visit as she could manage. It was emotional, but Lynn held her feelings together until the drive home, when she just could not contain them any longer. Her mum sat with her while she sobbed. There were no false reassurances of, 'You'll feel better soon . . .' or 'It will hurt less by . . .' What there was, though, was a silent acknowledgement that an event as joyful as the birth of a child could reopen a partially healed wound; and a grandmother who was willing to quietly sit with that pain.

For any family member or friend wanting to support a grieving family there will be times when you feel that you are getting it wrong, or that you just do not know what to do. Acknowledge that if you can and try again. Talk with parents about what might be needed, and most importantly of all talk about the child who has died. Often people make the mistake of avoiding mentioning that person's name or of reminiscing about the child. I have never come across a bereaved parent who has complained about how much people were talking about their son or daughter. Always the complaint has been that he or she is not mentioned. We sometimes avoid talking about the person who has died as we worry that it might upset the bereaved, but they are, of course, upset, whether we talk about the child or not. In *Continuing Bonds: New Understandings of Grief*,[1] Klass writes of one mother who said that her child's name may bring tears to her eyes, but music to her ears. In the majority of situations parents are desperate to talk about their son or daughter, as it is one way of keeping their memories alive. And who better to have these conversations with than family and friends who also knew and cared about the child.

Do not expect, either for you or for the grieving family, that once you and they are through the first year things will necessarily improve. Second years are hard too. There is no fixed time line for grief and many parents will say it can take three or four years before they begin to feel remotely like themselves again. Some of the most infuriating questions for bereaved parents are those containing the words 'still' or 'yet', some examples being: 'Are you still going to the cemetery every week?', 'Haven't you cleared his clothes yet?'. Those kinds of questions carry a negative judgement about the pace at which things are moving and are likely to receive a testy response.

Other major sources of irritation and upset are any suggestions that the child's death is 'for the best' or that they have 'gone to a better place'. No matter how much you think it might be true, comments about time healing will also be unwelcome. For recently bereaved parents, what they will be aware of is that each day that passes takes them further from that time when they last held or touched their child.

This is also not the time to suggest thinking about having another baby. Parents often hear that as a suggestion that someone else can replace the child who has died. As any bereaved parent will tell you, there is never a replacement and the majority will resent the implication that this will make them feel better.

So what can grandparents and other family members and friends do? The most important thing is to remember that you cannot take away the pain. Try to understand some of what is involved in the grieving process and take care of yourself. If you live close enough by offer to help with practical things, and if there are surviving children try to be there for them. Be sensitive to the difficulties which family events, even celebrations, may now create, and understand if the grieving parents cannot take part. Allow yourself to be human and recognize that you will not always do or say the right thing, but do the best you can.

Things to Remember

- This is not something you or anyone else can fix
- Recognize your own grief and get the support you need
- Talk about the child and share your memories
- Try not to make any assumptions about what the bereaved parents might need or want
- Most importantly be there and continue to be there

Reference

1. Klass, D. (1996). The deceased child in the psychic and social worlds of bereaved parents during the resolution of grief. In: *Continuing bonds: new understandings of grief* (ed. D. Klass, P.R. Silverman, and S.L. Nickman), pp. 199–216. Taylor and Francis, London.

Your Notes

Chapter 6

Anniversaries, birthdays, religious festivals, and family celebrations

Parent's Perspective

Tom died just two weeks before his thirteenth birthday and so I really didn't have time to register how I would feel about marking his birthday without him being there. His funeral had only taken place the week before and his grave was still covered with flowers. I decided to take up the offer from a friend to go and spend the weekend at her house, and so Charlie and I fled. I couldn't face spending the day either alone at home or with my family. With hindsight, I think it was exactly the right thing for us to do. There was no pressure to do anything other than surround ourselves with our memories and be gently looked after.

As the months passed, the whole subject of Christmas began to loom. I had absolutely no idea what I wanted and so allowed Charlie to make the decision for us. In the past, I had always had a big, traditional family Christmas—noisy, food-oriented, and hectic. It was always held at our house as it was equipped for Tom's needs and was just easier for us. When I asked Charlie what he would like to do, he didn't hesitate in stating that he wanted it to be like before. I felt very strongly that I didn't want Charlie to think that I couldn't be bothered to do things for him. I would have hated him to look back and perhaps think that he wasn't worth it.

The anticipation of the event itself made me nauseous, but I managed to keep myself occupied, and planned and shopped as usual. On Christmas Eve, Charlie and I went to the children's carol service at the church where we had had Tom's funeral. I had kept in touch with the minister who had conducted Tom's funeral and she gave us a star tag to remember Tom with and hang on the tree in the church. I enjoyed the anonymity of being a stranger there as it was a different church from the one we had normally attended at Christmas with Tom. It was hard going back into the chapel for the first time since the funeral, and I sat there in a complete daze, allowing the service to wash over me almost unnoticed.

We returned home and probably did a few last-minute jobs, including putting Tom's Christmas stocking on the foot of his bed. I have done this every year since as I couldn't bear to leave it in the box of decorations.

The following morning, we met with my family at the cemetery to lay flowers at Tom's grave. My tears did not hesitate to flow and I felt overwhelmed with grief. At this time, there was just a stark wooden cross to mark the grave and a patch of bare earth: my grief felt like the grave looked, fresh and unhealed. There was nothing anybody could say or do to comfort me. I just wanted to make sure Charlie was close by me. We eventually drifted back home to try and carry on as normal.

At one of the bereaved parents' group sessions that fell shortly before Christmas, we were each given a candle in a votive that we were encouraged to light at Christmas to remember our children. As a group we decided to each light our own candle at midday so that as it burned we could think of each other as well as our own children. This has now become an annual ritual and a candle has pride of place on my fireplace.

Our Christmas dinner table was usually set for twenty people and I cooked the usual feast. As soon as I sat down to eat, though, I knew that I just couldn't do it. I literally couldn't swallow the food. I excused myself and went upstairs to my room and just lay on my bed. I asked to be left alone, reassuring everybody that I was alright, that I just needed to spend some time on my own. Although Tom never sat at the table with us to eat (he was tube-fed), his absence was just too much for me. I allowed the quiet of my bedroom to wash over me and let my anxiety subside. When I eventually returned downstairs, other than a few surreptitious glances from my nieces and nephews, things just carried on as before.

The rest of the day passed, and I recall that the following day I felt unwell. Both Charlie and I had had a chest infection in the days leading up to Christmas and it were as though I had been given permission to now succumb to feeling unwell. It was the first time I had ever had such an illness, and I believe it was directly caused by the stress I felt at the anticipation of Christmas.

I didn't send any cards that first year as I couldn't bear the pain of not writing Tom's name on them. I was oblivious to any feelings that anyone might have over not receiving a card, and yet was horrified at the jolly festive messages that came my way in those that I received. I didn't even put them up but just left them in a pile on the table where my distaste was allowed to fester every time I looked at them. It felt as though people had quickly forgotten. I was so furious, that on our second Christmas I signed every card from Tracy, Charlie, and remembering Tom. It felt full of spite and I wanted to shame everyone in their omission of his name. It certainly didn't make me feel any better for doing it, but I still posted them all out! It felt totally out of character to me to do something solely with the intention of hurting other people's feelings, but I felt I had to challenge the world to understand who and what I had become. It made sense to me the following year when I attended the Service of Remembrance at Great Ormond Street Hospital when the minister read out a quote from another bereaved parent. He said 'You don't ever get over losing a child. You just learn to behave in public'. This resonated profoundly with me and made me think back to my behaviour in sending out those cards. It also made me smile! Ha! I was allowed to be badly behaved!

The way I have got around this problem of leaving Tom's name off any cards that I have to send is to put a rubber stamp on them instead. I bought a little dragonfly stamp and this has become my way of remembering him as always being part of our family. I'm not sure if everyone knows that this is my intention but it has become our family signature.

Our Christmases since have followed the same pattern: I continue to entertain my family at home after our morning visit to the cemetery. I find a certain amount of comfort in the familiarity of this tradition being carried on and I always remember how much Tom loved a big celebration.

Over the following years, on Tom's birthday, I have held a small family tea party with cake and balloons. I think the younger members of our family have enjoyed me still including Tom in the yearly birthday celebrations. I know that they love letting off a brightly coloured helium balloon into the sky each year (Fig. 6.1). I think that the adults secretly enjoy this too! As the years pass, I still feel a very strong urge to mark his birthday, to keep him as part of the extended family.

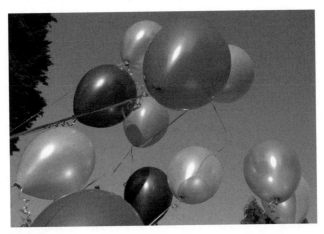

Fig. 6.1 Balloons.

The year at the time of writing (2011) would have been Tom's eighteenth birthday. I decided to arrange a meal out to mark this milestone. I felt an enormous need to celebrate and remember Tom on this significant birthday. I toyed with the idea of doing something at home but made the decision to let others do the work for me so I could relax amongst friends and family. We went to a restaurant that I had often taken his carers to for our Christmas meal, so it held some fond memories too. Everybody thoroughly enjoyed themselves and we toasted Tom after my sister made a short speech. It was noisy and fun and he would have loved it! My eldest nephew insisted on buying champagne and I know Tom would have been delighted. I also think this meant a lot to Charlie, as he looks up to his cousin, in a way, as a big brother.

Celebrating my own birthday is another time when I often feel overwhelmed with my grief. As I mentioned in Chapter 1, in the first year my birthday was very soon after Tom had died, but subsequent years have probably been sadder. I find myself feeling very low and out of sorts for the day, at my most reflective. When I have days like that, I tend to allow myself to just go with it, and it actually revitalizes me now to be given the time to remember Tom and sit quietly, perhaps listening to some music that we both loved or being out in the garden.

Easter is always a particularly difficult time for me because it was on Easter Monday in 2006 that Tom became ill for the last time. As ever, as a family, we always celebrated Easter with a big gathering and usually an Easter egg hunt. It was one of Tom's favourite things—to hold the basket that the other children would bring their eggs to during the hunt. He absolutely loved it, to the point that we often had to re-hide the eggs so he could do it all over again. He usually held on tight to the basket for the rest of the day, thrilled at having been given such an important job!

On Tom's last Easter we were in the garden and I noticed that he didn't seem too well, and over the next few days his chest became worse and worse. Easter Monday, therefore, remains a significant day for me too but without the added stress of having a particular date associated with it as Easter obviously falls on different dates each year.

Mothers' Day is also difficult for me. The first year, it felt so incredibly wrong to first take flowers to the cemetery and then to take flowers to my mum. Charlie always signs my card from both him and Tom, which I love, although I have to confess to being terribly upset the first time. Not so much from what was written; more that Charlie had actually made the decision himself with no prompting.

The anticipation of the first anniversary of Tom's death was a hugely anxious time. I had recognized that it would be from early on and wanted to mark it in a special way. As I mentioned in Chapter 3, Charlie and I spent time in the lead-up to the anniversary arranging for Tom's headstone to be made. It was one of the cemetery's regulations that you could not have a permanent headstone for twelve months after a burial and so I made it my mission to have one by his first anniversary. I wanted it to be a surprise for everyone and so we kept all the details a secret. All our plans worked out and it was erected a couple of days before. I did have to request that nobody visited the cemetery in the week leading up to his anniversary as I wanted to 'unveil' it to everyone on the day. I also asked Jan, our minister, if she would bless the stone and so we had a little gathering at the cemetery that day. I requested that Charlie had the day off school and it was one of those surreal days when I just felt as though I was living in slow motion. Everybody loved the headstone and Charlie and I were thrilled to show it off after all our hard work!

Reaching the first anniversary of Tom's death was a huge milestone. I remember being so conscious of having to describe the time passed since him dying in years rather than months. Similarly, in the early days, it was difficult changing my language from weeks ago to months ago. Reaching the New Year had this impact too, when I had to change from saying that Tom died this year to last year.

Each year now, on his anniversary, Charlie and I visit London Zoo. The first year we decided to become Friends of the Zoological Society of London which gave us unlimited admission to both London Zoo and Whipsnade Zoo. We joined in memory of Tom, who loved all animals and loved going to the zoo. I still request that Charlie has the day off school, as I think it is an important date for both of us and one that the school should respect. I am not sure for how long Charlie will want to go to the zoo, although I am hoping that for him, like me, it is a place he will never tire of.

I would like to share here something that happened this year (2011). At the end of 2010, Buckingham Palace announced that Prince William and Kate Middleton would be getting married. The proposed date happened to be Tom's anniversary. I was devastated. It felt so, so wrong. Particularly when it was then announced that there would be a bank holiday to mark the occasion! As the date approached, Royal Wedding fever hit the country and it seemed that every shop and newspaper had my special date emblazoned all over it. I felt violated! I wasn't sure if going to the zoo would be an enjoyable experience given that London would be full of people, and then fate dealt us a hand: my youngest nephew gained a place in a diving competition in Sheffield on that weekend and so we decided to travel up with him and not go to the zoo that year. It seemed like the perfect excuse not to have to sit through the television coverage of the wedding as we were on the train at the time! Not very patriotic, but hey! It was actually nice to be able to spend the day with Charlie and his cousins on a little adventure. The day had a bit of extra significance as it was Tom's five-year anniversary. Five years seems to be another milestone, for some reason, as I'm sure ten years will be too.

Professional Perspective

Life is never the same again after the death of someone you love, and sometimes these changes are unexpected. Significant family events and dates take on a whole new meaning in the aftermath of a loss. While grieving, events that had previously been celebrated may be transformed into bittersweet or downright painful occasions. Your son's or daughter's birthday, which previously may have been a source of great joy and anticipation, may now be tinged with or completely overwhelmed by sadness. Other family members' birthdays, including your own, may, for a time, feel like something that has to be endured not celebrated. Religious festivals—Christmas, Eid, or Hanukkah—will also be changed, as events which were once eagerly anticipated become yet one more thing to get through. You will also have to face the anniversary of your child's death. You may find that other associated dates weigh heavily too. These might be the date of your child's diagnosis, the decision to terminate treatment, or of a significant hospital admission. Holidays will also be altered. Some families recognize that they can perhaps travel to places which previously would have been impossible, but many of them would willingly give that up to have their child be with them for one more trip.

The ever-present awareness of the loss of your child is all the more evident on these significant dates and events, so emotions will be heightened at these times. Added to that is the anxiety that is felt as families anticipate these occasions and wonder if, or how, they will cope with them. I sometimes remind families that these feelings are normal and also that many of them had the same anxiety about, for example, the funeral, or returning to work, which, with support, they managed. And, as if the awareness of the loss and worry about coping is not enough to handle, you also have to juggle your partner's or extended family's expectations of these dates. Surviving children, unless they are adults, will in all likelihood want and expect Christmas and birthdays to continue to be celebrated as before. This means that you will have to manage your own feelings, anticipatory anxiety, and others' expectations around all of these events.

How do grieving parents manage all of this? What I have seen work best for a lot of families is to acknowledge that the event is approaching—ostrich behaviour does not work here—and to make a plan for it.

Remember, too, that ultimately anniversaries and birthdays are days like any others and what helps you generally will work on the 'special' days, too. If you are approaching the first anniversary, birthday, or Christmas remind yourself that other parents have got through this and in many cases the hardest part is the anticipation, not the day or event itself.

Having a plan can help in a couple of ways. It allows you to take control, which is a step towards managing the anxiety that comes with the anticipation. It also helps you get through the day, partly because of the preparation it requires you to do. Developing a plan forces you to think about what is important to you, what might feel right, and, equally importantly, it helps you to identify what you do not want. You will also have to think about how your needs and expectations will sit with what other family members are hoping for. Two parents I worked with viewed their son's birthday very differently. For Edward's mother it was important that while she knew she would be sad, she also wanted to celebrate the life Edward had had and the happiness his birth had brought. For her the first birthday after his death had to include balloons and a home-made cake. Edward's dad did not feel able to celebrate, but did not dissuade his partner from doing what was right for her—and he did manage to eat some of the cake. Even though they chose to spend the day privately, both parents were heartened and felt supported by the friends and grandparents who acknowledged the date with cards and letters.

In my experience there is a vast range of ways in which families choose to honour both birthdays and anniversaries. I have seen families who essentially want to close the door on the outside world and remember very privately. In contrast, I have also known parents who threw birthday parties and invited everyone. One family planned a special service at their local church, at which they celebrated the life of their daughter, Freya, with music, readings, tributes, and laughter. A number of families have planned birthdays and, less frequently, anniversaries as family days out, engaging in an activity which their child enjoyed. Andrew's family always marked his birthday with a train ride, as this had been one of his favourite things to do.

If you have children of school age, talk with their teacher about difficult dates, especially if you are planning to take your child out of school for the day. Every year Hamish's parents plan a family day out on the birthday of his sister, Naomi. In the first couple of years this was met with surprise by school staff, but in Year 2 his teacher suggested that he make a digital album of photographs, recording the day. The family did this and Hamish then had the chance to show them to his class during 'Show and Tell'. He was proud to talk about Naomi and even took questions from the other children about how his sister had died, which he handled brilliantly. His parents feel this was an important milestone for him in telling his story at school and gaining respect for his experiences.

Anniversaries are painful days and again there is no right or wrong way to 'do' them, but a broad spectrum of possibilities. Some families will choose to return to a significant place to mark the day. At Helen and Douglas House families sometimes request to visit the hospice on the anniversary or to spend time in the grounds. For others that is too painful to contemplate. Many families spend time at the graveside or where the ashes are buried or have been scattered. They might do this individually or as a family. Often they choose to do something symbolic such as sending off Chinese lanterns or writing messages and inserting them into helium balloons, before watching them float off into the sky.

Whatever you choose to do, talk about it with your immediate family and try to accommodate each other. The majority of parents plan to take the anniversary, and sometimes birthdays too, as leave from work. As mentioned above, many will also take siblings out of school for the day. If you decide to take a day off work or take a child out of school it is a good idea to be honest about what the time is for. You may not be at your best in the lead up to these dates or for a little while after. If your employer or child's teacher understands what is happening, it is more likely that you and they will be supported.

The extended family may well take their lead from you. If you want privacy let them know that. Equally, if it is important to you that family and friends acknowledge these dates, whether you want them there in person or would prefer cards or letters let them know that, too. They are more likely to get it right for you if they know what you need or expect. Remember that they cannot be mind readers. As their son's anniversary approached one couple sent emails and cards reminding friends and families of it and sharing their plans for the day. Letting people know what you need will save you from feeling hurt, angry, or disappointed after the event.

As I mentioned earlier, having a plan can be enormously helpful, but I always remind families that a plan can be changed or abandoned all together if it does not feel right on the day. Remember, too, that the choices you make about the early birthdays and anniversaries are not set in stone and may change as time goes by. For one family the idea of Christmas at home without their lovely daughter was too much, and for the first few years after her death they always arranged to be away. More recently though they have begun to spend Christmas back in their own home and now it feels the right place to be.

Anniversary reactions are not uncommon around landmark dates. They may last only a few days or run into weeks, and you may find yourself re-experiencing some of the early feelings of grief as well as mentally reliving the events of your child's last few days or hours. Freya's anniversary is in mid-December, but from the middle of November her mum relived the changes in her daughter's condition and her increasing care needs leading up to her death. Over the years since Freya died, her mum has come to recognize the timing and pattern of her feelings. This has meant that she can plan around them. She has learned, where possible, not to schedule anything too stressful at this time and she also knows, from experience, that the feelings change as the anniversary passes.

We have talked so far about significant dates which are personal to you and your family, but we know that shared events and celebrations will have an impact too. Religious holidays and other annual events can be painful as well. Mothers' Day and Fathers' Day will be especially poignant without your son or daughter, but you might also find that less obviously emotional days will unsettle you too. These could be seeing your child's peers transfer from primary school to secondary school or from there to work or university. Attending the wedding of one of their friends may also be a bittersweet experience.

One of the biggest challenges for families is handling the big religious festivals. Even non-Christian families can struggle with Christmas, as it is such a significant part of life and culture in the UK. While you can perhaps shut out the world around birthdays and anniversaries, it is almost impossible to shut out Christmas and other people's excitement and anticipation.

Family traditions at this time of year have very often been passed from generation to generation. Whichever religious festival you observe, some of the celebration relates to a sense of belonging and to being part of a family that is unique and special. We all accumulate memories over the years and typically look forward to the next festive season. When someone close to us has died, that anticipation becomes clouded. We watch as those around us prepare with excitement and our grief may be intensified. Acknowledging your anxiety about the coming events can be the first step in managing it. There are no definitive ideas on how best to handle this time of year. What follows, though, are some suggestions, drawn from the experience of bereaved families themselves.

Acknowledge your emotions—tears, sadness, anger, or anxiety are very normal reactions and you do not have to pretend that they do not exist. Grief will not go away because it is the festive season, indeed, if anything, it may intensify.

Think about what you can comfortably handle and let others know what that is. Rather than focusing on other people's expectations, do what feels right for you, even if it means letting go of past traditions or things you feel obliged to do.

Let others know whether you want to talk openly about your son or daughter, or not. If you normally host the celebrations, think about whether you want to continue to do so this year. Are there ways in which others could help or take over this responsibility?

Some people have found it can be helpful, or make things less painful, to do things differently. These changes can be small or fairly major. You may consider going away somewhere different for Christmas or New Year instead of staying at home or visiting relatives. As well as the family I mentioned above I can think of many others who, especially in the first year, have escaped to somewhere without any memories or connections to their child, and also where no one will have any expectations of them.

Families who have stayed at home have found it helpful to open presents at a different time or to eat at a different time. Another possibility is to have friends or family take over some of the things that you or your son or daughter has normally done.

When it comes to buying gifts, it may be easier if you have a list and do it on a 'good day'. Remember, though, that even good days can have their difficult moments. If you think it will be easier, try shopping with a friend who understands or accept offers of help and let friends do your shopping for you. You can, of course, do a lot of it from the comfort of your own home, especially using the Internet.

Some families have chosen not to send any cards at all, at least for the first year. If you do send them, it can be hard to decide on how you want to sign the cards. Many parents find it impossible to think about not including their son or daughter's name. One option is to sign it, and add 'in memory of . . .' or 'remembering . . .'. Tracy's suggestion of a symbol representing your child on the card is also a good one. You may find it easier to take some time and decide how you want to sign the cards before you actually sit down to do it.

Many families feel strongly that they want to acknowledge and remember their child at Christmas. There are a number of ways to do this. You may think about adding a new tradition or ritual, for example visiting the cemetery or a special family place at or close to Christmas. Sometimes the symbolism of lighting a special candle in memory of your son or daughter can be helpful. In some of the support groups at Helen and Douglas House parents have chosen a particular time on Christmas Day at which they all light a candle, allowing them to remember not only their own son or daughter but also the children of the parents they have come to know from the group. One couple I supported who decided to continue their tradition of spending Christmas with their own parents took their candle with them and asked family members to join them in lighting the candle and remembering their son. You can also remember your child with a favourite flower or plant to have in your home, or take to the grave. Another option might be to choose or make a special ornament or decoration for your tree or for your home.

For some families it seems quite wrong not to be buying a present for their child or young adult. If you feel this way, you could consider giving a gift in memory of your son or daughter or donating the money you might normally spend to a favourite charity. Buying a living Christmas tree or plant to put in your garden might be another option.

When you are thinking about what to hold onto and what you can let go of, these questions may be useful:

+ Have I considered other close family members' expectations and told them what is important for me?
+ Do I or other family members really enjoy doing this?
+ Would Christmas be Christmas without it?

Finally, remember that the Christmas season is stressful for everyone. Grief is exhausting and when combined with that time of year it can be particularly difficult. Exhaustion alters perception and can make things seem worse, so make sure you have enough rest and ask for support when you need it. If you do manage to enjoy any of the celebrations, allow yourself to do so. It does not mean that you have forgotten or that you are betraying your son or daughter. And keep in mind that whatever you choose to do one year may not be what you decide to do the next year.

Thing to Remember

+ Recognize that birthdays, anniversaries, and other celebrations may intensify your grief
+ Think about what will be important for you to do
+ Check how your partner or children want to mark the occasion
+ Let the extended family know what you need or want from them
+ Recognize that the days leading up to the birthday or anniversary will probably be more difficult than the day itself.
+ Remind yourself that what helps you on normal days will also help you with the significant dates and events

Your Notes

Chapter 7

Getting the support you need and what to do if it lets you down

Parent's Perspective

I can be completely categorical about how to get support: join a bereaved parents' support group! It may sound like the most awful thing to want to do when you are feeling so bereft, and I can, without a doubt, say that the first time I attended a workshop at Helen and Douglas House I had never felt more nervous. When I have talked to other bereaved parents who have not had support from such an organization, their initial reaction has been one of not feeling able to do such a thing. I will be honest and say that it is an emotional experience (obviously), but the benefits far outweigh the initial discomfort of being almost open to the elements about your experience.

Over the last five years, I have created what I like to think of as a toolkit of coping strategies for my bereavement. There are many things in there that I have gleaned from real-life experiences or, perhaps, things I have read and made a note of when they have particularly resonated with me. Often, as with my twenty-minute strategy that I talked about in Chapter 1, they have come from completely unexpected sources. By actually writing them down (I tend to use a notebook app on my phone, which is always with me and therefore instantly accessible) I find that I have been able to look back over them and re-affirm their significance. Things such as poetry or lines from a book all have a place in my notes as a permanent reminder of their importance to me.

My first venture into getting support was a visit to my GP within the first eight months after Tom died. Both Charlie and I had been unwell with a persistent cold and chest infection. Added to the physical feeling of being low, were the emotions and mental feelings that were exacerbated by it. I remember talking to my doctor about the possibility of getting some support and was more or less told that there was a very basic service for counselling in my primary care trust and it wouldn't necessarily be pertinent to bereavement. I was also offered the choice of whether I wanted antidepressants. At that stage I felt quite sure that I would not want to go down the route of pharmaceutical intervention. I came away from that appointment feeling deflated and with an overwhelming sense of having to get on with it by myself.

The following January I decided to see a homeopath as I was having some problems sleeping. I had an excellent recommendation for a lady called Felicity and my first appointment was, in my opinion, a huge success. The whole ethos of homeopathy is to treat the whole person, and after a long discussion with her about my background and experiences, she decided as a starting point to treat me for shock. This made absolutely perfect sense to me, and I felt physically lighter at the prospect of doing something positive about the way I was feeling. I felt that by looking at the root cause of my grief, and of course the whole of the nine years that had preceded it, I could really begin to find myself on the path of learning to live with it.

Alternative medicine is not for everyone, but I had always been open to other ideas and taking a holistic approach was something that I had always advocated with Tom. I visited Felicity every month for the rest of the year until she took a sabbatical. Having the space and time to talk to her about the way I was feeling was just as important as having the remedies she gave me. Of course, it helped that we gelled immediately and so I felt completely at ease talking to her. Over the course of that year, I tried many remedies but should confess that my sleeping pattern remained largely unchanged! What I can recognize, though, is that by having the chance to be proactive about the way I was feeling was the start of what I consider my journey through my grief.

On the subject of alternative medicine I also read up on crystal healing, and I am rather partial to being surrounded by beautiful crystals! I wear a wonderful ring with a large rose quartz set in it that is my constant reminder of the power of love, whether it be romantic love or familial love, and I always think of my boys when I look at it. Rose quartz is said to be a powerful healing crystal and so I am willing to take all offers! The point I am trying to make is, that if something makes you feel as though you are actively doing things that you find are giving you some comfort, just do them! I liked reading about the healing properties of my crystals; I liked to read that someone, somewhere believed that they had qualities about them that might make me feel better. Simply put, I just liked to see the words grief and heal together in the same sentence, in black and white, rather than just inside my head.

Ten months after Tom died, I had a letter from the bereavement team at Helen and Douglas House inviting me to attend a workshop for bereaved parents entitled 'Do men and women grieve differently?'. It felt as though it came at just the right time. I had had a couple of sessions with Felicity and so had begun to get used to opening up about how I was feeling. Even so, the thought of going alone to a place I had only been to once before, and not knowing a single person there (staff or parent) was extremely nerve-wracking. I decided to telephone them and ask for a bit more information and whether I could bring someone with me for moral support. I was told that as the group was specifically aimed at bereaved parents, it would be inappropriate for me to bring somebody who wasn't bereaved themselves. I then took a deep breath and confirmed that I would be attending.

My drive to Oxford that day had me in a highly anxious mood about what I was about to encounter. I really needn't have worried. I was met and welcomed into the group, and after having a cup of coffee and a friendly chat with a couple of people about things totally unrelated to my bereavement, my nerves began to disappear. Once everybody had arrived, we sat in an open circle and were given the opportunity to introduce ourselves. I can't quite remember whereabouts in that circle I was but I clearly remember being overwhelmed with the honesty and openness of its members. When it came to my turn, I gave my name and a few brief details about Tom and how he had died and, with that, my tears started to flow. For the first time, I felt I was in a safe enough environment to allow this to happen.

I wasn't offered platitudes, I was given the space to allow my grief to take on a physical manifestation. I knew I was in a place where I didn't need to find words to explain how I was feeling. The sense of sharing was huge and long overdue. I didn't have to wear a mask or pretend everything was all right. Over the course of the workshop I was encouraged to participate as much or as little as I would like. Other than the introduction, there was absolutely no pressure to contribute vocally, and I soon learnt that I could get just as much from attending if I chose (for whatever reasons) not to actually say very much at all. Being a listener was just as valuable, and on more than one occasion that was all that I did—listen to what others had to say. It is hard to say what reasons I had for choosing, on occasion, not to talk very much. It could have been that other things were bothering me more at the time or even that I had had a bit of a tricky journey getting there. Whatever the reason, I was never made to feel as if I was less than part of the group.

The morning went by very quickly and I realized that by lunchtime I was starving! I always smile to myself when I think back to all the lunches I have shared at Helen and Douglas House and how we have all devoured the food put in front of us! It is as though the opening up of our deepest emotions is hungry work! The other thing that became obvious after the very first meeting was that it was also exhausting. This was something that we had been made aware of previously, and after the first workshop I remember feeling absolutely shattered for about three days afterwards. As I began to participate more, I tried to make sure that my diary was clear for at least a couple of days afterwards as I knew I wouldn't be up to speed as a result of the emotional significance of sharing.

At the conclusion of that very first workshop, I was invited by the bereavement team to join a parents' support group. It would consist of about twelve bereaved parents and we would have to commit to a block of meetings spread over the following eight months or so. I decided to join, and our initial meeting was just a few weeks after that first workshop.

The group sessions were, without a doubt, where I can say that I finally began to find my way forward through my grief. Again, our first meeting was very much in the vein of introductions and getting to know one another, but having already experienced this, I was much less anxious. Having said that, my tears and emotions readily welled up. I consider it a huge privilege to have been part of such a close-knit group who have all shared such deep feelings. Unusually, I think, everybody in my group had lost a son and it seemed to make a difference to us in our bonding. We would refer to our lost children as 'our boys' and it enabled us to feel like a very tight-knit group. Spotting the similarities between our boys, be it an identical article of clothing or favourite toy, was an unexpected bonus of our time together.

The group meetings had loosely woven themes or topics for discussion, but we were never made to feel as though they had to be adhered to and we went off on many tangents! A common part of each meeting was to spend five to ten minutes having a one-to-one discussion with the person sitting beside you, each taking it in turns to speak for the allotted time. This made it possible to get to know and share details of each other on a more personal basis. I found it particularly enlightening talking to the male members of my group, as I felt that I was completely unaware of how men grieved.

Each group meeting was eagerly anticipated by me and we were all sad to see it coming to an end. We tried to keep the group going for a while, and we did manage to meet a couple of times, but life seemed to get in the way and so unfortunately the opportunities dwindled. I have often met up with members of the group at other workshops and remembrance days at the hospice and it is clear that we formed a very strong bond that is unlikely to be forgotten.

To people who have never lost a child, I have found it has seemed a very odd thing to do—to spend time talking about children dying. This just goes to show that the needs of bereaved parents are still very misunderstood and the whole subject is still almost taboo. I certainly didn't ever really discuss with my family or the majority of my friends what is was that I was finding there at the hospice. My bereavement often felt like an incredibly lonely journey, and these sporadic meetings were a source of companionship and understanding.

I remember meeting up with a mum I knew from Tom's school who had lost her son shortly after Tom died, and I told her how much support I had found at the hospice and that perhaps she would benefit from something similar from the hospice that she had used for her son. She showed a lot of reluctance and I wished I could have been more persuasive because I can wholeheartedly say that it was the thing I found most beneficial during my grieving process.

This difference in needs between people who have shared similar experiences is a really important thing to remember when you are on this journey of grief. I have learnt from the other parents I have talked to that there is no right or wrong way to grieve, and what might work for one will not necessarily work for another. I have found that the sharing of experiences has helped to broaden my outlook on the world as I found it when I was ready to emerge again.

That first workshop at Helen and Douglas House also brought about another equally important part of my rehabilitation. I was offered individual support from Christine. It was exactly what I had been looking for in my unsuccessful conversation with my GP a few months earlier. At first I was so surprised that the hospice was willing to take me under their wing, so to speak, as I had never actually used the hospice with Tom. We had gone through the referral process and had got as far as trying to plan a weekend there for respite but, as things turned out, we never made it and I had already decided that I would not want to use it for end-of-life care for Tom. To be picked up by the hospice's family support and bereavement team was an unexpected gift.

I hastily planned a date for Christine to visit me at home on the back of what I felt was such a successful day at the workshop. I had witnessed the relationships between members of the team and the other parents in the group and it became clear that I would benefit from such support. For so many months I felt as though I had no adequate words to describe how I was feeling, but when Christine and I first met I began to formulate the thoughts and find the words to work my way through the jumble of feelings and emotions that I was finding increasingly difficult to unravel.

For the first time I felt as though I was in a safe enough place to say what I needed to say without fear of judgement or pity, and slowly found myself able to find ways of making sense of the plethora of emotions that were crippling me. We talked for many hours over the next two years, when Christine would pay me a monthly visit. I never imagined I had so much to say! Being given the chance to talk openly was a new concept for me and one that, if I'm honest, took a little getting used to. I was always amazed at how quickly the time passed when we were sitting around my kitchen table! I appreciated being given the chance to be listened to and gently persuaded to question and sort through the difficulties I was experiencing. I was able to admit that quite often I was not 'fine' and that sometimes I found wearing the mask of 'I'm fine' intolerable. I was able to express my frustration at the unhelpful comments of other people that I had to experience on a fairly regular basis.

I should mention here that dealing with other people, whether they are friends, family, or total strangers, can be a very daunting task. People are often at a loss as to how to respond when they have been told that you have lost a child, and I have often then found myself being in the position of the one having to do the comforting when the other person is clearly upset or uncomfortable with the information they have just been given. For that reason, another useful tool to have in your armoury of coping strategies is one where you make an often split-second judgement about how much information you should give out about your circumstances. Equally, it must be said that sometimes it is just as hurtful for no acknowledgment to be made at all. I have spent many hours talking about this particular subject with other parents, and although we have been able to express our anger and frustration, we have also been able to laugh about it. A sense of humour is, to me, an essential part of my toolbox, which probably sounds like a complete oxymoron to apply to a bereaved parent! I think that many parents who have or have had a sick or disabled child will be able to resonate with this fact, and I can recall laughing along with my group members at some very black humour that would not dare show its face in conventional society!

My time with Christine gave me the opportunity to work through the different stages of my grief and the different obstacles I seemed to encounter along the way. Without offering me solutions, she guided our conversations towards self-discovery where I could learn to accept things or make an active choice to try to accommodate how I felt my life had now become. Our conversations touched virtually every aspect of my life, and although there are some things that remained unresolved I can take comfort from the fact that it wasn't for the lack of trying!

I have often been asked if I have ever sought a medium or psychic, and this has been discussed many times within the workshops or groups I have attended. It is something that I think is a natural thing for a bereaved parent to consider but personally I have never felt the need to go down this path. It could be that I am cynical or it could be that I simply don't believe. Without sounding too airy-fairy, I have at times felt a certain presence of Tom around me and this has always been enough for me to take comfort from without attempting to find more concrete evidence of an afterlife. Many parents with whom I have had conversations have shared that they have their own personal signs or happenings that they like to think of as being connected to their child. Mine has always been a white feather. The rational side of me tries to scoff at the mere idea of a feather floating down from seemingly nowhere at pertinent times, but the softer more gentle side of me always smiles inwardly as though it is perhaps our little secret. A little sign to say that he is still with me. If I am away from home, it has become a little ritual that, all of a sudden, a white feather will appear from nowhere and I will acknowledge it and say hello! I do recall finding it quite unnerving being told that Tom had made an appearance in another parent's time with a medium. I felt almost violated for some reason, and angry too. Not so much that I had not experienced it for myself, rather that, even in death, other people were intruding on our relationship.

An opportunity that I did not hesitate to take up was the invitation from Helen and Douglas House to attend a spiritual retreat. It was held in a beautiful house of a benefactor of the hospice and run by Mark, the then chaplain, and the bereavement team. At first I felt a little unsure about the significance of what I considered to be a religious retreat but was assured that I could participate as much or as little as I felt comfortable with. The first one I went to was arranged into group presentations focusing on art, music, and poetry.

The first group presentation was based on Michelangelo's Pieta sculpture. Mark talked about this image and how it represented loss. I found it incredibly powerful to see Mary cradling the body of Jesus in her arms. It resonated with me in a way that words cannot describe. I think the image will stay with me forever. Mark talked about a sense of holding on and letting go. It is a feeling that I am aware of now in my life as I move on into territory that is new and challenging.

It was at the first spiritual retreat that I was made aware of the book *The Spiritual Lives of Bereaved Parents* by Dennis Klass.[1] Excerpts were read from the book during the day and I decided to buy a copy for myself. It is not the easiest of books to read because it is quite academic, so I knew it was not going to be something I would read from cover to cover. I have picked it up many times over the years since I bought it and am always grateful that I have because there have been words in it that have made absolutely perfect sense to me. Klass talks quite early on about the reaction of people to the thought of going to a bereaved parents group and describes one man as responding that he attended 'because once in a while it is nice to feel like everybody else'. This was another affirmation that although the way I was feeling often did not make much sense to me, I knew that I was not alone. I even found an almost perverse kind of comfort when I read that Klass considers parental grief to be a permanent condition. Reading that made me feel that there was no rush to feel 'better'. It was another discovery that I added to my toolkit to help me to accept the way I was managing my grief.

I have always felt quite in awe of the parents who I have met who have found such a lot of comfort from their faith. I have never been a particularly religious person, and since Tom first became ill when he was four years old I have questioned the whole religious element. I have had to listen to others expressing their opinions about whether there is a God if children are allowed to suffer and die. The thing that I consider taking away with me from the retreat days is that faith has many guises and having faith in yourself is an important asset to have—another tool for the toolbox, but a difficult one to come to terms with sometimes.

I chose to have Tom's funeral service in a church, so deep within me there is obviously a need to respect the faith I was brought up in but in which I have never fully participated. I feel fortunate to have formed a friendship with Jan, the minister who took the service; she has been a part of my support system ever since. We have discovered that we share many interests, and when we meet it is not necessarily in a spiritual capacity (for me) but I have always taken comfort from the prayers we have shared together.

Jan gave me a book called *Bread for the Journey*[2] for Christmas in 2007 that was described as a yearbook offering short spiritual reflections for each day of the year. I started reading it on the 1st of January and, as prescribed, read each morning. Some of the pieces were short and took mere seconds to read and others were longer and required deeper thought. One of the passages that touched me deeply was for January 2nd! It talked of joy and sorrow being our spiritual parents. This had never felt truer to me. I have never hesitated to recommend that bereaved parents (or anyone else for that matter) read this book because it was such a gentle, positive gift.

The Klass book, along with the retreat days, also made me take a broader look at what I thought about living a more spiritual life. I found comfort in reading that one could lead a spiritual life that was not necessarily religious. This made perfect sense to me, because the experiences I had had previously that could possibly have come within the realms of religion had had the opposite effect on me and made the void seem even bigger. My idea of religion was to feel part of a community and that wasn't necessarily something that I believed had to be done in church. The feeling of community at Helen and Douglas House was exactly what I had been looking for.

Later on, in 2007, I started writing a blog. At first it was just general thoughts and sharing of ideas in a predominantly craft community but it slowly opened up into a whole range of topics that I felt I wanted to record and share and eventually I wrote about Tom and my grief. As I began to form relationships with my readers, my feelings of finding a new place to be were being compromised by not talking about the most important part of my life: that of one without Tom.

I was sent this beautiful poem by one of my blog readers in a private email after I had posted about Tom's birthday one year and I would like to share it here as a message of hope:

Hold On To What is Good, a poem by noted American poet, Nancy Wood

Hold on to what is good
even if it is
a handful of earth.
Hold on to what you believe
even if it is
a tree which stands by itself.
Hold on to what you must do

even if it is
a long way from here.
Hold on to life even when
it is easier letting go.
Hold on to my hand even when
I have gone away from you.

I am still writing (albeit mainly nonsense!) to this day, and have gained so much from finding myself in another community that has nurtured and fed me via cyberspace. It seemed to be a win–win situation for me. I could get into the habit of writing regularly, I was being inspired on a daily basis, and I found I was capable of forming new friendships in a place where I felt I belonged—a little like the parent groups but in a totally different context. I choose not to blog about Tom very often but my blog gives me a much-needed personal space to record the things that I felt were significant to my life and wove them through everyday life and they remain a permanent record of how my life has panned out since he died. Writing is very cathartic and it is another thing I would wholeheartedly suggest doing. Words, either on paper or on a screen, are much more powerful than the maelstrom that tends to form in your head!

Professional Perspective

In the days, and perhaps weeks, after your son or daughter dies you may well feel overwhelmed by the numbers of friends, family, colleagues, and casual acquaintances who call by, write or phone, and offer their condolences or practical help. You would not be the first family to have a freezer full of lasagnes and every vase in the house full of beautiful flowers. But what happens when the flowers have wilted and the food has been eaten? For some parents that initial outpouring of support continues and families feel held and supported. Others find themselves in a situation in which both emotional and practical support decreases.

In a crisis, as a death is, people will go the extra mile to be there for you, but often what is forgotten is that for you the crisis continues beyond the first few days and weeks. Friends and families may step out of their normal life and routine for a short time, but soon both work and family life claim them back. This frequently coincides with the initial shock and numbness wearing off for you. You therefore find yourself facing the reality of what has happened just as the calls, visits, and offers of help taper off. At this point you will have no idea for how long you will continue to feel tearful, angry, or vulnerable, and your support network may not have a clue either. What I have learned in supporting parents is that very often there is a discrepancy between how long it actually takes you to feel emotionally stable again and how quickly friends and family expect you to reach that point.

In Chapter 5 I mentioned the danger of 'still' and 'yet' questions, and I think they are worth repeating here. They are one of the biggest bugbears for parents in terms of other people's understanding and they might sound something like this: 'Haven't you cleared his room yet' or 'Are you still not back at work?'. Implied in the 'still' and 'yet' questions is that there is a timeline for grieving and sorting things out, which clearly the parent is not meeting. Friends, family, and people in your community may have expectations of how you should be managing this, and what I regularly hear from parents is that these expectations are completely unrealistic.

Where do they come from? Conventional wisdom says that in the wake of a loss the first year is the hardest. Facing all the firsts—birthdays, anniversaries, holidays etc.—without your child is, undeniably, diffi-cult. What can be forgotten, though, is that it does not magically become better once you have done that and there can be an expecta-tion that once you live through the first year it should be business as usual. That may sound fine to someone who has not experienced a significant loss, but in practice it does not come close to the truth. Parents often tell us that, in fact, the second year is harder. So there is a confusion about what is a realistic period of grieving. Alongside this is the heartfelt desire of family and friends to see you 'well' again. That is for two reasons: firstly a genuine concern for you and the pain you are in, and secondly it is hard for them to see you experience that pain. If your suffering decreases or disappears altogether, then some of theirs will too.

This mismatch of expectations can create real tension. I can safely say that I have never been in a support group with bereaved parents in which the issue of family and friends' lack of understanding has not come up. Sometimes, as a facilitator, one wonders who these people are and what they can be thinking about, but often, even though their attempts to help may be clumsy or miss the mark, they do usually come from a place of good intentions. It is easy to write off inept family members and friends, but some context may allow us to understand them, if not to excuse the mistakes. Most of us simply do not know how to talk about death and we are acutely uncomfortable with this topic.

As part of induction training for new staff and volunteers at Helen and Douglas House we would include a language exercise. Trainees would be divided into groups and given five minutes to produce a list of as many words and phrases as possible for death and dying, which would then be shared in the large group. This apparently light-hearted task always produced an enormous list of descriptors, which would include gentle euphemisms, humour, and some pretty harsh lan-guage. There were many serious teaching points to be made from this, but what is relevant here is that the plethora of language we have for death does not actually mention death itself and is an indication of our discomfort with the topic. Most people lack an appropriate vocabulary with which to talk about it. Your friends and co-workers may want to ask you about how you are feeling but they will not necessarily know where to start. And the passage of time seems to make this more difficult. Meeting a parent shortly after the death or coming to the house specifically to offer help seems manageable. Bumping into that same parent six months later appears to leave people tongue-tied and awkward. Should they acknowledge the recent loss or ignore it? Should they mention the child's name or should they even talk about their own children? If we listen to bereaved parents the answer is obvious; of course they should, but there are people who will have no idea of where to begin. In every support group we have heard of people crossing the street to avoid talking with one of the bereaved parents. Thankfully this behaviour is the exception, rather than the rule, but it is painful nonetheless.

What can you do when someone is getting it wrong, whether with an insensitive question or an incorrect assumption? You have two options. You can say nothing or you can explain what is happening to you. Saying nothing may be the easy option—in the short term. It avoids any uncomfortable conversations, but leaves you feeling hurt or disappointed and if your friend or colleague does not know that he or she is missing the mark he or she will continue to do so. If you explain, for example, that repeated questions about when you are going back to work are not helpful, then it is less likely to happen again. More importantly it also creates an opportunity to say what *would* be helpful. A gentle reminder to a family member that when you are upset all you really need is to be heard and perhaps held could save you from some unhelpful platitudes about it 'being for the best'. A further consequence of saying nothing is that you begin to withdraw from people. You might think what is the point of spending time with someone if you come away from it feeling worse? The danger here is that you compound the isolation that we know grief brings and you add to the feeling that no one understands. Sometimes people will need help to understand. They will take their lead from you. If you talk about your child it lets them know that it is OK to do so. I always think that this is an unfair responsibility to put on bereaved parents, but if you do not try to help people understand what is going on for you there is a good chance that they will misread you and misunderstand what you need and want.

Saying nothing also means that you will increasingly be forced into situations where you have to behave in ways which show nothing of how you are really feeling. Numerous parents have talked about 'putting on the mask'—by this they mean that they put on a face to cover the pain inside. If a neighbour in the street asks how you are, what they expect to hear is 'fine' or 'OK'. They are not expecting to hear how hard it was for you to even get out of bed that morning. Parents rightly feel they have to do a lot of masking of their true feelings just to survive in everyday situations. Tracy, in an earlier chapter, talked about not getting over losing a child but instead learning how to behave in public. Do you really need to 'behave' with everyone? If you feel you cannot be honest with close family and friends, then when and with whom can you be yourself?

If you think you are not receiving the help you would like from family and friends, or you decide that you do not want to burden them with how you are feeling, what choices do you have? Most children and young adult hospices will have a family support or bereavement team, which will offer either one-to-one support or perhaps a group with other parents. If you have not previously used the hospice it may still be worth making contact, as some will also take clients from the local community. Organizations like Compassionate Friends and The Child Bereavement Charity can also help. We talked about bereavement support earlier in the chapters on couples and grandparents. Sometimes parents ask, 'What good will support do—it won't bring my child back, so what is the point?'. Clearly it will not bring back your child, but it can make a huge difference to talk with an independent person, who will neither be afraid of your feelings nor tell you how you should be grieving. Grief support, either individually or as a couple, can help you understand what you are feeling and also help you recognize the strengths you are tapping into in order to live through this time. Even with amazing family support there may be things which are just too painful or personal to talk about with them. A bereavement counsellor or support worker can be that sounding board for you.

One of the lessons learned over the years at Helen and Douglas House has been the enormous value of bringing bereaved parents together. Whether in an on-going group or a one-off workshop, sharing with other parents decreases that sense of isolation. Parents often describe groups as the one place where they can remove their mask and not feel that pressure to 'behave in public'. They share what is working for them as well as what they are finding hard, and as a group they learn with and from each other. Most importantly they support each other. Talking with another parent about their experience of a difficult sibling or the first anniversary can help you come up with ideas to manage your own situation.

Sometimes parents are reluctant to join a group. When you are already sad, you may ask yourself why you would want to spend time with other equally sad people. What is surprising about the groups is that while there will be sadness and tears and anger there is also a lot of laughter. Yes, it is hard to come into a room full of strangers and talk about your child or to hear other parents talk about theirs, but what typically develops is a strong support network and people who stay in touch way beyond the relatively short (six sessions) life of the group. At Helen and Douglas House one of the unintended outcomes of the groups is that families also support each other when they come back to remembrance days. When they are coming for the first time it seems to be easier if they know that some of the members of their group will be there. One parent described his group as 'the club no one wants to belong to', but its members were relieved to have found each other and to know that they could count on each other.

The workshops combine more recently bereaved parents with those further along in their grief. In meeting parents for whom years have passed, the more recently bereaved see living proof that the pain changes and that people survive this. And sometimes too it is in spending time with those earlier in their grief that the more experienced parents are reminded of those early days and recognize the progress they have made in incorporating their loss into their ongoing lives. In short, parents give each other hope.

Sometimes it is not from people that we derive support or energy—instead there are beliefs which sustain us or activities which we know will replenish us. You may find comfort in your own beliefs, whether they are religious or more broadly spiritual. We ran occasional workshops on spirituality at the hospice which generated a lot of interest, and parents' definitions of what spirituality means to them have been diverse. It is striking, though, how many parents have spoken of feeling their child's presence around them. Tracy talked about the significance for her of a white feather. For other parents it is a particular bird or butterfly, sometimes even a fox, which they experience as a link with their child. Some parents have consulted mediums but others would never dream of doing so. Dennis Klass has written in detail about parents and spirituality in his book *The Spiritual Lives of Bereaved Parents*,[1] discussed by Tracy. As with *Continuing Bonds*,[3] his writing is grounded in parents' experiences. One of his suggestions in the book is that the deceased child becomes a force for good in the parent's life. This really resonated with parents who came along to the spirituality workshops and with those who have read more of his work.

For the introverts among you, your energy may come from more solitary activities which allow you to reflect and re-charge. Time spent alone is no bad thing. You may find that a walk in the woods, a swim, or a yoga class replenishes you more than a conversation about what you are truly feeling. From time to time Helen and Douglas House has run a one-day retreat for parents, which Tracy has described attending. These days were the opposite end of the spectrum from the groups and workshops as the focus was on reflection and quiet time rather than on talking and listening. Parents used the day in different ways. Some came to the optional input sessions where we used art or poetry or music to help people focus and reflect. One mum spent the day curled up in a hammock in the beautiful garden, while another brought a box of photographs of her son, which she carefully sorted and admired. Parents left with a sense of peace and expressed how luxurious it had felt to have time and space to think about their son or daughter without any distraction. Of course, it is not necessary to attend an organized event for this. You can create your own reflective time within a solitary activity, which you enjoy.

When you can summon up the energy, creative pursuits are also sustaining. Something I admire in Tracy is how creative she is, and when I visited her I was always curious to see her quilting, her stained glass, or her photography. I knew that whatever creative project she was involved in, and usually there were a few on the go, it was an integral part of her support system. Some of her activities she pursued in isolation, but some brought her into contact with other people—in person and on-line. As baking is another aspect of her creativity, it was also a treat for me as her bereavement counsellor to walk into the house and smell freshly baked cookies or cake!

Getting the support you need requires you to have some sense of what it is that sustains you and also know who can help. Sometimes the knowledge is already there. You may have already learned that you are someone who needs space or someone who wants to be surrounded by family. You may know who is good at helping with practicalities but runs a mile when you show any emotion. Take a look at your friends and family. Think about what you might need and who might be able to provide it. If you cannot face the school run or football coaching is there a friend or family member who can do that for you? Is it a different person who can sit with you while you cry or rant and not try to close you down or falsely reassure you that it will all be fine? If you have no energy for cooking or housework are there friends who can do it for you? What you need will change over time as will who might be best to help you. Allow yourself and your support circle to change. What has worked for you in other difficult times may need some adjusting. Recognize that while some friends will let you down, there will be others who will step up and surprise you. Perhaps one of the biggest obstacles to finding support is allowing yourself to accept it. No one can fix this for you, but you do not have to manage it on your own. Assume that if people offer to help they are sincere in that offer, and then accept it. Give yourself permission to be supported!

Things to Remember

If you find you are not getting the support you would like:

- Clarify for yourself what is missing
- Conserve your energy for the things that matter to you
- Allow others to help when they offer
- Keep a list in your head of tasks that others can do for you and when people ask if they can do anything, offer them something from your list
- Let friends and family know what it is you need from them (and also what you don't . . .)
- Don't limit your support to people. Think broadly about what helps you through the day or night

Things to Remember *(cont.)*

- Don't isolate yourself
- Think about some bereavement support or counselling
- Find a bereaved parents' support group—contact your local children's hospice, Compassionate Friends or The Child Bereavement Charity

References

1. Klass, D. (1999) The spiritual lives of bereaved parents, 1st edn. Routledge, London.
2. Nouwen, H.J.M. (1997) *Bread for the journey: a daybook of wisdom and faith.* Harper Collins, New York.
3. Klass, D. (1996) The deceased child in the psychic and social worlds of bereaved parents during the resolution of grief. In: *Continuing bonds: new understandings of grief* (ed. D. Klass, P.R. Silverman, and S.L. Nickman), pp. 199–216. Taylor and Francis, London.

Your Notes

Chapter 8

Medical questions and concerns

Parent's Perspective

Within a few weeks of Tom dying, certain aspects of what had happened began to play on my mind. When there is seemingly nothing else you can do except sit around all day feeling totally lost, it seemed that constant questioning and playing back of recent events was inevitable.

One of the most notable thoughts that kept recurring was the weight of having had the sole responsibility of administering certain medicines to Tom in his last days, without a professional in the house.

Shortly after Tom died, there was a lot of media coverage about the aftermath of a hurricane in the United States. I read of doctors and other emergency professionals being heavily criticized for making decisions about who should be saved in the immediate state of emergency. I read with horror that it was being suggested that some people were being given drugs to quicken their expected death so that the medics could concentrate on the ones who would survive. They were the very same drugs (particularly morphine and midazolam) that I had had responsibility for giving Tom to make him comfortable in the last days. I kept thinking that maybe I had actually killed Tom instead of allowing him the dignity of dying naturally at home. These thoughts were persistent and plagued huge chunks of my waking hours. I became increasingly worried that, to some, I may be thought of as a terrible mother.

I decided to take up the offer from Tom's paediatrician that I could make an appointment to go and see her if I needed to. I voiced all my feelings about what had been going through my mind and she assured me that I had done absolutely nothing wrong. I had used my judgement as to when Tom needed drugs such as the morphine and midazolam, following from the years of experience I had had with managing his illnesses and his disability. I had been fully supported in my wish to have Tom at home and as far as everybody was concerned I was competent to achieve this. I remember her explaining to me that she had heard similar thoughts from other people in situations like mine. I was able to express the weight of the responsibility that went alongside carrying out Tom's end-of-life care. It was such a relief to be able to talk about it to someone, as I felt completely unable to voice how I was feeling to anybody for fear of judgement. I was anxious about whether the members of my family who had been at our house when Tom died may have had the same thoughts about me too. My mum and sister, in particular, were always very questioning about the care, and especially the medication, that Tom was given. I felt a huge burden of shame while my thoughts went down this path.

Throughout Tom's short life, my way of handling difficult situations with the many medical concerns that I had was to try to gain as much information about them as I could. I was never afraid to ask questions and I had to remember that it was just as important to apply this strategy after he had died. I recall that when Tom first got ill, when he was four years old, I asked why it was that he had become so severely and critically ill when the majority of people would have had much, much milder symptoms. I will never forget the consultant explaining to me that some children who got chicken pox got maybe four or five spots, while other would be simply covered in them. It didn't really explain the actual reason but it put it into a perspective that I could at least begin to understand. With hindsight, I can recognize that this explanation was a foundation stone for my levels of acceptance of what had been dealt to us. The question 'why?' is so often the first on parent's minds and it is without doubt the most difficult to answer.

In the months leading up to Tom's death, there was a lot of discussion about his end-of-life care. I was encouraged to ask as much as I liked about any aspects of this as I felt necessary. To start with, my questions were very basic: I had seen a dead person before (my grandmother), but I still felt unprepared for what death would actually be like. I needed to know *exactly* what would happen. I needed to know the process of death. I needed to know what I should do if Tom died, for example, in his sleep and I found him the following morning— who should I call? What should I do? Of course, nobody could give me any actual answers, but the opportunity to have a frank and honest discussion was a hugely beneficial part of my coping strategy. I also found that I needed to repeat many of the same questions in order to allow the information to settle within me. I believe that there is a certain amount of shame in being ignorant about death and its manifestations. When it is your own child who is going to die, this shame feels incredibly debilitating and it is extremely difficult to overcome. I can recognize that it was the safe environment and established relationships that I had created with the professionals in our lives that allowed me to admit to my need for information on such a distressing subject.

When I discussed Tom's prognosis with my GP, she informed me that from that point on she would see him every two weeks as a matter of routine. At the time, if a child had been seen by his or her GP within two weeks of their death there would not have to be a post-mortem. Again, I felt grateful for this proactive approach by my doctor to avoid further pain and distress. More often than not she would call in on a home visit on her way to the surgery in the morning while Tom was getting ready for school, creating the least disruption possible. It was gestures like this that, again, made life just a little easier to come to terms with.

I feel incredibly fortunate to have benefited from the experience of the wealth of knowledgeable professionals around me at that time who could advise and support me over all the worries I had. A huge concern of mine before Tom died was that he would be taken ill at school or elsewhere outside the home and would be taken by ambulance to an unfamiliar hospital. When I mentioned this, I was relieved to hear that a memo could be placed against his name at the London Ambulance Service with a directive about his care. It was stated that I was to travel with him (they needed to wait for me to reach him) and that we would go to our local hospital even if it was not the nearest. Things like that made a massive difference to me. It felt as though I was being considered as an important player in the chain of possible events. Likewise, that Tom would be comforted that I would always be with him.

Another issue that was raised was the possibility of Tom being resuscitated. Again, I had discussed this at length with our paediatrician and we had come to the conclusion that it was not appropriate for this to happen. Tom's respiratory function was already compromised and the chances of him recovering from being extubated were very slim. I certainly had no wish to be in the position of deciding when to stop life-support. Likewise, if the need arose for him to have further intravenous antibiotics this was not considered to be in his best interests regarding his quality of life, particularly because he was already taking prophylactic antibiotics.

I made the decision in the process of this planning not to share all the details with many people. Being divorced from John, meant that I attended Tom's hospital appointments on my own and so there came a time when John had to be involved in the discussion as he still had parental responsibility. In spite of having an amicable relationship, there was little communication between us about the children and I felt dreadful about having to broach the subject of Tom's prognosis with him. Once again, our paediatrician stepped in to help and so an appointment was made for both of us to attend her clinic.

It was incredibly difficult to have to sit in on the conversation that ensued, as John had almost walked in blind to what he was about to hear. When I had arranged the appointment I had given him some warning about what it was about but I can appreciate how hard it was to hear news like that for the first time from medical professionals. Being emotionally distant, there was little we could do to comfort each other and I felt as though the void between us was completely unbridgeable.

I then had to make Tom's school aware of how things were, and I remember feeling particularly judged when I met with the head teacher and other members of staff at school. I do not really know why it was such a strong feeling other than that I felt that my relationship with school was not especially strong as Tom had not been there for very long. I had always felt that the way Tom and I did things was a bit different from what they were perhaps used to. This was often a feeling I experienced from having a child with an acquired brain injury rather than a child who had been disabled from birth. It is a very complex experience having watched a perfectly healthy child become one who is so hugely dependant, and I often felt that this was a massive part of the way I learned to live with such an experience. I was already living with a feeling of loss, and so for the rest of Tom's life there was a precarious balance of feeling grateful that he was still alive coupled with the ongoing difficulties we now had to face.

It was also distressing to tell his carers who worked with him at home. I had a wonderful team of women who were devoted to Tom and I knew they would be very upset at the news. It was important that they knew what to do if things suddenly became serious, and so I had to share with them the protocols that had been put in place. I also felt compelled to give them the option of thinking about whether they could continue given the circumstances, as I knew that it would be very upsetting. Of course, they all stayed!

My GP encouraged me to share the burden of what I was carrying with someone within the family and so I decided to tell my sister. It was a very difficult decision to keep the rest of the family out of the loop as it were, and my reasons for doing this were very complex. Part of me did not want my parents, in particular, to have to worry about us. Over the years I had developed my own coping strategies, one of them being to offer only as much information as I could deal with being known. With the information, came much questioning and opinions and I just felt that I could not support anybody else's distress at the time. I felt that as I was the one who was Tom's primary caregiver, no one else would ever really see things from my own perspective, regardless of how much they might try. I wanted people to act normally around us and to give me the opportunity to act normally around them. I didn't want all my thoughts and worries spilling out into every aspect of my life—it was more than enough having to carry them around with me constantly anyway. Being able to compartmentalize was crucial to me managing my concerns. I felt that I had lived in a goldfish bowl for many years with having to have so many people involved in our lives, that this was a very private time for me and I did not want it to be part of an open discussion.

Professional Perspective

At Helen and Douglas House we have supported families who have experienced a sudden death as well as those for whom the event may have been anticipated, if not quite expected at the time that it happened. That means that we have seen families with long-term diagnoses, some whose children have died after a relatively short illness, and some families for whom there had never been the certainty of any diagnosis at all. In each category parents are often left with questions about their son's or daughter's illness and its treatment or management. With a sudden or unexpected death, parents may be completely bewildered by what has happened. It is hard enough to take in medical jargon and explanations in the best of circumstances and when you are reeling with shock not much of that information is retained, far less understood. After the initial numbness wears off you may struggle to make any sense of the medical background to your son's or daughter's death.

Early on in bereavement support visits I have repeatedly heard parents talk about the events leading up to their child's death and also describe in detail the death itself. There is a sense in which the telling and re-telling help make what happened real for people. Alongside the need to go over what happened, there are the questions parents ask of themselves, such as 'Did I do everything I could?' and the related question as to whether the medical team also did everything it could. Those queries may relate to preventing the death, but equally may refer to whether the child was as comfortable as possible, with pain well managed.

For some families these questions are either dealt with fairly easily or may fade into insignificance, but for others they can grow and even begin to become an obsession. Some of the more painful emotions of grief may be displaced. Consciously or otherwise it may be easier to be furious with your child's doctor or the hospice or hospital staff than to acknowledge your fury that your son or daughter has been taken from you.

The need to understand is multilayered. In addition to trying to make sense of those last hours, days, or weeks, you may have questions about the health of your surviving children and children you may want to have in the future. These can be particularly pressing when your child's condition was undiagnosed or had a genetic component.

If the questions are growing or causing you serious concern, make an appointment to talk with your child's primary doctor, explaining what the purpose of the meeting is. Just as you will need to prepare for this appointment, this allows the physician to do likewise. Prepare a list of questions you would like to discuss and take it with you to the appointment. Parents do not always agree on the need for or value of this kind of consultation, so do not be surprised or angry if your partner is reluctant or simply does not want to participate. If it is important for you, though, go ahead and do it. If you are not going with your partner, take someone with you whom you trust. Two pairs of ears are better than one, and if you become upset you may want your support person to ask the questions for you. You may also consider asking the doctor if you may record the conversation. Trying to absorb important information in a stressful situation may mean that you miss significant aspects. A recording will allow you to hear it again when you are calmer and perhaps less distressed.

Once you are in the appointment, take the time you need to work through your questions. Ignore any concerns you have that you may be bothering the doctor. I cannot think of one instance of a family going back to see the medical team when they have been dismissed or not accorded the time they needed. If you need further referrals, for example for genetic counselling, talk this through and ask your doctor to arrange it for you. If the idea of returning to the place where your son or daughter was treated or died is too much for you, ask whether a home visit is possible. Su Laurent, a consultant paediatrician at Barnet General Hospital, north London, is very encouraging of doctors making home visits for these conversations.

If you have older surviving children they may want to be part of this process. In fact in one family I supported it was the teenage siblings who initiated the medical meeting. Sara, struggling to make sense of her sister, Jamila's, end-of-life care, emailed the hospital team asking for some answers. In response the family was offered and took up the opportunity to meet with the staff involved. This case is a good example of parents having different needs. Sara attended the appointment with her brother, Samir, and her mother, Lisa. Sara's dad felt that as no conversation would bring Jamila back, he did not need to be part of it. The outcome of the meeting was that the family understood more than they had before, even if it did not completely resolve their concerns. They were, however, heard and taken seriously. While it is unusual for the children to initiate the medical consultation, you might think about asking your children what questions they would like to have answered. At one of the Helen and Douglas House sibling groups we arranged a question and answer session with one of our palliative care doctors. Much of what the children wanted to know about was how their brother's or sister's condition might affect them: 'Will I get sick, too?', 'Will my children also get muscular dystrophy?'. This might mean that you go to your appointment with questions about the past, i.e. what happened to your son or daughter who died, but also about the future and what the implications might be for your surviving children.

Over the course of a lifetime with a sick child parents have to become expert advocates; negotiating care packages, benefits, and educational provision. I have sometimes wondered if there is a degree to which these post-death consultations are a final act of advocacy on their son's or daughter's behalf. They may also improve practice for other children and families. When they think things may have been done differently, parents usually feel strongly that the care staff or doctors learn from this and that other children and families benefit from their experience.

For many families who go back to the medical team these consultations often take place within the first year after the child has died. However, that is not always the case. Kim requested a consultation with hospice doctors four years after her daughter, Bethany, had died of cancer. She thought she had understood and accepted the decisions made about her daughter, but after seeing a television documentary in which someone with a similar diagnosis had a very different outcome, she began questioning her daughter's treatment and the decisions which had been made. After a conversation with one of the doctors Kim realized that not only were the two situations different, but that treatment options were constantly changing and developing. The 'Should I, or could I, have done something different?' question may have a different answer as treatments change and improve. While it is distressing to learn that advances in medicine might possibly have resulted in your son's or daughter's life being extended, you have to remind yourself that the decisions made and the resulting outcomes, good or bad, reflect the circumstances and the knowledge of the time. Most discussions I have had with parents in relation to treatment or end-of-life care decisions ultimately come to the conclusion that parents have made the best choices they could with the information they had at the time.

Earlier in the chapter I mentioned the need to understand your child's medical condition or cause of death, particularly in relation to any thoughts you might have about future children. It has been my experience that this can be one of the most agonizing decisions parents may have to make following the death of their son or daughter— whether to try to have more children or to keep the family as it is. Similar to many of the choices we have discussed in the book, there is no right or wrong outcome, only one that works for your particular situation and stage in life. Of the families who have gone on to have further children there is seldom any intention or hope of replacing the child who has died. The mistaken, but often given, advice about another baby taking away the pain of the loss does not generally apply. Tracy chose not to have another child, but we can take some time to look at two very different family situations, where the parents did have more children, and unpick some of the thinking that lay behind their decisions.

Holly and Pete were the parents of Edward, who had been poorly since birth but undiagnosed with any condition until just two months before he died, aged fifteen months. Prior to the diagnosis and his death, unaware of the life-limiting nature of his condition, Holly and Pete had begun to think about another baby. After Edward had died they were still considering another pregnancy. Although there were many pros and cons they were in fact reassured by their recent knowledge of the genetic condition as this meant there were tests which could be carried out, none of which would be definitive but which would allow them, along with the genetics team, to weigh up the risk of a future child having the same condition.

As a couple they looked carefully at all of the ramifications of trying to get pregnant. These included the risk of exposing themselves to further loss if, for example, Holly miscarried. They also had to think through the choices they may have to make if the genetic test results were ambivalent or indicated that the baby would have Edward's condition. Could they or should they go ahead with the pregnancy in that situation? They also thought about other people's reaction to another baby. Would family and friends think it too soon or a sign that they were 'over' Edward? Would people think of a new baby as a replacement for him? If they did manage to have another child, how would they feel about him or her using Edward's room, playing with his toys, or even wearing some of his clothes?

After much thought and discussion, they chose to go ahead and try. When, five months after Edward's death, Holly became pregnant, it was a time of mixed emotion. Their joy at the possibility of a new baby was tempered by anxiety as they proceeded through scans and tests. They were drawn back to memories of Holly's pregnancy with Edward and their feelings about it and saddened that he was not part of this experience, becoming the big brother they had hoped he would have been. It was not until around the fifteenth week of the pregnancy that they were told that the risks of this baby being affected by the genetic condition were small, and it was only at this point that they felt they could begin to relax a little and to start to tell people the news. Holly described herself from this point on as feeling 'cautiously optimistic', with her confidence growing with each further step. Her antenatal care was at the same hospital and clinic as it had been with Edward and sometimes it was hard to separate the memories and feelings associated with his development from that of the new baby. Attending antenatal classes was also a challenge and they found it a 'learning curve' as they had to respond to the very normal questions from other parents about whether this was their first time or if they already had children. These innocent enquiries can create a real dilemma for bereaved parents as they do not want to deny the existence of their son or daughter who has died and at the same time are concerned not to unsettle expectant parents looking forward to perfectly healthy babies whom they anticipate will outlive them.

Holly and Pete's pregnancy and delivery went smoothly and they now have not one, but two little girls. Holly describes them as having three children, but adds that they were 'childless for a while' (during the time between Edward's death and the arrival of the girls). That 'childless spell' was, in my opinion, pivotal in their and in other parents' decision to have more children. It is true that they were planning another child before Edward died and they were clear that it was not about replacing him. However, in that time without a child to physically parent, they realized how much being a parent meant to them. Many of the things we complain about as parents—getting up in the night, never having a moment to oneself, or being a taxi service—are the very things that bereaved parents would yearn to be able to do again, as well, of course, as all the fun bits. In Chapter 2 we looked at the issue of identity and the question of whether you are still a parent if your only child dies. That can be a real and relevant consideration in the decision to have another child or not.

Sally and Adam's experience is quite different from that of Holly and Pete, but there are a number of overlaps in how another baby changed life for them. They had two children, Luke and his older sister, Becky, who were both healthy, until Luke was diagnosed with cancer. His death at the age of twelve devastated the family. They have since had another son, Josh, and while they did not have to think about genetic conditions, it was not a straightforward decision for them either. Sally says that part of what drove her to think about another child was the awareness of the love she and they as a family had to give. She had been totally involved in Luke's care and was aware not only of the huge gap left in their life, but also of Becky's (appropriate) growing independence. In Sally's own words: 'It wasn't just having a lot of love to give that prompted the decision for another child. It was also the desire to be needed, especially as I had had three years of intensive looking after Luke. After his death it was so empty. Becky was pushing me away. Adam was busy trying to get his career back on track. I felt very alone, empty and just not needed.'

For this family a further significant factor in thinking about another child was the hope that something positive might come from the life they had had with Luke and the impact of his absence. They thought that a baby would bring hope and joy and something to look forward to.

Sally says they were 'older' parents when they first began to think about another child. They looked initially at adoption, ultimately deciding not to pursue that, not least because the agency would not consider them until at least two years after Luke had died. That, in combination with their age and the length of time it might take to adopt, meant that it was not the right option for them.

As with Holly and Pete, Sally and Adam's pregnancy was an emotional time for the family. Sally had similar experiences to Holly's of talking with other parents and answering the questions about their other children, but she feels overall that the pregnancy and now Josh's presence in their life have positively changed how their family relates to the outside world. News of the pregnancy was something positive to share and since Josh was born their life has expanded, becoming more social. Like many bereaved families they had become quite isolated after Luke's death. Having another child has seemed to free others to talk about their own children without feeling that they were being insensitive. People have begun dropping by again—especially Becky's friends—and the house is busier and livelier.

Holly and Sally chose to learn the gender of their babies during the pregnancy. Initially Pete did not want to know whether they were having a girl or a boy, but he did change his mind and asked to be told. He and Holly felt that it was positive that, following Edward, they were having a girl. Sally and Adam were happy to have a boy, who may or may not be like Luke. With hindsight what was clear in both situations was that the foreknowledge of the baby's gender and the time that allowed each family to adjust to the idea of having either a girl or a boy was hugely valued. Looking back neither would have wanted to deal with that 'surprise' at the birth, which anyway was enormously emotional.

As with any new baby, siblings can react positively or negatively, and of course it is often a combination of the two. For a bereaved sibling the birth of a brother or sister can raise questions about their own place and value in the family. Questions such as, 'Am I not enough for you?' or 'Will you still have time for me?' are not unusual. Sally dealt with these concerns by explaining to Becky that parents do not have a finite amount of love to give. The love she has for Becky is neither diminished, nor decreased by her love for Luke and Josh.

The families we have just looked at knew that they could continue to love their child who had died and to have space for other children too.

Sometimes parents feel that they could never love another child in the same way or that it would somehow be disloyal to have another child. One fear that is voiced both by parents who do have another child and those who decide against it is that there will be less time and space to think about and remember the child who has died. While the fear is real, forgetting a loved child is not something I have seen in families with whom I have worked. In fact, what each of these families has experienced is that their babies have connected them to Edward and Luke and provoked memories of them. Sometimes they have found that painful, and sometimes comforting.

In few situations will the decision about a subsequent pregnancy be a straightforward one. There may be medical or genetic concerns, as well as purely practical and emotional ones. On the informational side, do not be afraid to talk to your doctors, or where it is appropriate to ask for a referral to a geneticist or genetic counsellor. Ask for the information you need so that you can make an informed choice. It will be impossible to make a decision on medical information alone, but it may help you to clarify the choices you have.

Sally feels she is a more relaxed parent now and says she 'takes things day by day'. Here are her final comments on their experience to date: 'It [having another baby] doesn't take away the grief or what you've lost. It doesn't discount what went before. It gives a different perspective. It gives hope.'

To return to the broader issue of handling those medical questions and concerns, think of the people who have cared for your son or daughter as a potential resource. One conversation may be enough to set your mind at rest or to reduce the frequency with which your mind takes you back to distressing situations or scenes. Alternatively, understanding and making sense of medical issues may be a process. You may need to take in the information, bit by bit, allowing time to understand and assimilate it before moving on to the next phase of understanding.

Sadly, sometimes, there is no real explanation as to why things happened as they did. Just as some families have to live with the uncertainty of not having a diagnosis for their son or daughter, it is not always possible to adequately explain how or why a death occurred at a particular time. That level of uncertainty can be hard to live with and sometimes parents torture themselves with the 'not knowing'. Often, however, they reach a point where they feel they have to draw a line under it and live with what is, rather than exhaust themselves with either what might have been or what was not.

Things to Remember

If you are considering talking with your child's doctor or care team the following might be useful:

- Make a list of questions to which you would like answers, or issues that you have not understood

- Make an appointment with the doctor and let him or her know in advance what you want to discuss

- Take the time you need in the appointment and don't feel rushed

- Take someone with you—two pairs of ears are better than one

- Try to have realistic expectations about what can be achieved

- Consider questions about the past—what happened with your child—and also about the future—issues for surviving children or relating to future pregnancies or children

Your Notes

Chapter 9

Planning a funeral

Parent's Perspective

Tom's funeral was something that, given his prognosis, I was able to think about and tentatively plan before he died. For me, it was another thing about which I could make some thought-out choices rather than it being a potential last-minute panic. I was very mindful that it would be the last thing I could do for him. It used to bother me terribly that I could be thinking of my child's funeral while he was still alive, but I believe this goes to show the way my level of acceptance was colouring my view of our situation.

Because I had already discussed with our doctors what would happen when he died, I had an idea of some of the things that needed to be done. Of course things never go exactly to plan; because Tom died on a Saturday night preceding a Bank Holiday that in itself presented some delay in organizing the funeral. I had a gut feeling that I didn't want there to be a long stretch of time before the funeral as I knew that this would be very difficult and stressful; I have since talked to other parents who chose to delay the funeral of their child for a variety of reasons and with hindsight wished that they had not.

I had to wait until the Tuesday after Tom died to do anything practical and was advised by our funeral director about the process. I was fortunate in that our funeral director was an old family friend, and this seemed to make the experience so much more personal to us because she knew both Tom and me. In fact, I had had the opportunity to talk to her before Tom died to get some idea of what would need to be done. As with most other things in my life, I had certain ideas about things!

After Tom died, I knew that I would have to get a doctor called out to give me medical certification of the cause of death so that I could register it. This took place in the middle of the night, and was one of the worst experiences I had to endure. I was enormously distressed to have to witness this as it felt like a very final thing. I then arranged for the undertakers to be called to take Tom to the funeral home. Having been so upset at the doctor coming, I made the decision not to see Tom leave the house with the undertakers. This was one of the very few times I took a back seat.

I remember going to see the funeral director first thing on the Tuesday morning and going over the procedure. The first thing to do was to register the death. My sister made an appointment at the registry office and I recall that it was a very dignified procedure and, unexpectedly, not hugely emotional. I think that this is because of the overwhelming professionalism of the registrar. Platitudes were kept to a minimum and it felt as though it was an unpleasant but necessary task. We were provided with the death certificate and the correct documentation for the funeral to go ahead. I find having both Tom's birth and death certificates together in a folder incredibly sad.

Armed with the paperwork, we could now go back to the funeral director and organize the funeral itself. I knew that I wanted Tom buried and so that was the first thing that the funeral director organized—the burial plot and arrangements with the cemetery. As we went along, she kept us informed of the costs. The majority of funeral directors do not charge for children's funerals but there are some costs incurred that have to be paid, particularly the cemetery costs. It seemed awful to have to talk about money at such a time.

We had been tentatively aiming at having it on the Friday of that week, which did not leave us much time to make the necessary arrangements. I'm guessing that something within me kicked in and I found myself in organization mode again. Once the date and time had been confirmed with the cemetery, the funeral director very much led the way with what else I needed to consider. The first thing was a coffin. I knew in my heart that it seemed wrong to have a big heavy wooden coffin for Tom and a long-ago stored memory of more natural caskets came to the front of my mind so I asked about the possibility of having something a bit more like this for Tom. I ended up choosing a beautiful woven bamboo casket that I felt was so much more appropriate for my gentle son. I knew that I wanted it adorned with natural-looking flowers and not contrived wreaths.

I would really like to stress the importance of taking your time and talking about the things you want for a funeral, as it really did make the difference to the day for me. For some reason, although I found myself baulking at traditional elements of funerals, I had a real bee in my bonnet about the funeral cars! I had an almost ridiculous hatred of those newer models of hearses that I had seen around and insisted that I wanted an old-style hearse and cars and not a Volvo. To me, it felt somehow more respectful. I wanted to try to make sure I could look back on the day with no regrets about the details of it, and moreover that it would reflect the life Tom had had.

I came away from the funeral directors that afternoon feeling quite satisfied that everything would be as I wanted it. I knew exactly what was left to be done. Charlie had suggested that he would like to release a white dove at the graveside and this was arranged by the funeral director too. I will always hold in my mind's eye the sight of the dove flying up into a cloudless blue sky that day and of Charlie's face as he released it. He was nine years old and more grown up then than ever and I was bursting with pride but overcome with sadness.

The funeral director had contacted the church where the service would be held and so Jan, the minister, telephoned me to arrange a convenient time to visit to discuss the service and find out a little bit about Tom so that she could prepare her own reading.

By the time Jan came to visit, I had had offers from my sister and two close friends to do a reading at the service. I was so pleased as I knew that I would be unable to speak myself. It soon became clear that there would be many people attending the funeral and I felt that I wanted it to be a true celebration of Tom's life. Jan also helped me choose hymns and music for the church service and advised me on the practicalities such as parking and seating arrangements.

Over the following couple of days I hastily accepted all offers of help as I felt I was in a tenuous state of control. Charlie and I went to the florist and chose flowers for Tom's casket and Charlie also wanted some sunflowers from him. I had shared with the people who were going to come that I wanted family flowers only and that donations could be made if they so wished to The Children's Trust where Tom had had his rehabilitation. I think this is a much more beneficial thing to do than have a field of flowers go to waste, and knowing how the money people donated was eventually used is a very fitting memorial to Tom.

We also had to think about what to wear, and that meant a frantic dash to try to find something. I had also decided that I didn't want people to wear the traditional black or dark, sombre clothing so I didn't stress about finding something that I wouldn't normally wear. I loved that Charlie said he would like to wear Tom's boots for the funeral. Looking back, I think it is wonderful that Charlie wasn't afraid to say what he wanted and hope that he can look back on the day as one where his involvement was very important.

Another thing that I was gently advised to consider was to get someone in to help with the 'reception' at home following the service and burial. As I said earlier, I already had an idea that there would be a significant number of people attending and so, on a recommendation, I found a local catering company that could provide some refreshments and a light lunch. I also accepted the offer of a neighbour to be at the house while we were at the funeral and let the caterers in to prepare the buffet and then let guests in as they arrived.

I also readily accepted offers of help to come and do some cleaning and general tidying up. Not that the house was in a state, more that things had obviously slipped over the previous weeks. It sounds ridiculous, but at the time these things really mattered to me. I felt conscious that I would very much be the focus of attention and this made me feel very uncomfortable. Several times over the course of the afternoon of the funeral I took myself off for some private time in my bedroom, as it was at times very overwhelming and excruciatingly tiring. Of course there were also a lot of people attending who I had not seen for a long time, so there was an awful lot of catching up to do with some of them who had been shocked at hearing of Tom's death.

Another aspect that was extremely important to me in the planning of Tom's funeral was that I was very aware that there would be quite a few children there. Besides Charlie, there were another eight children in Tom's immediate family, plus lots of friend's children too. I didn't want them to be more intimidated than necessary by the whole affair, and certainly not to be frightened by what might happen. I wanted them to be allowed to remember Tom and be glad that they had had him in their lives. Later on in the afternoon of the funeral when I glanced down the garden to see them playing on the swing and being boisterous (which included some scrapping!) I felt relieved that they were comfortable at least, even if some of them were probably too young to understand what was really going on.

The following day, I went back to the cemetery and took some photographs of the flowers and tributes and also to collect the cards that had been left. These, along with my sympathy cards and letters, are now stored in a box and I have often spent time poring over them and re-reading the words of comfort to be found there. When I read of how much support and love Tom received during his lifetime from people it fills me with hope that he will continue to be an inspiration to others as he was to me.

When I think back to the day of the funeral itself, I am satisfied that it was the best I could have done for Tom and that it was a day that reflected his life as best it possibly could. There were pieces of his favourite music, an abundance of family and friends, and a good measure of chaos thrown in, even if it was just the sheer numbers! Tom loved the hubbub of family gatherings and parties, and I like to think that he was looking down on us all and having a little wobble of glee as was his wont.

It is standard practice, I believe, for most cemeteries to have a period of a year before you are able to install a headstone. Planning the headstone would, I felt, be the last thing I could do for Tom, and as I discussed in Chapter 3 Charlie and I spent months deciding what we would like to have. As time has passed, I find I don't visit the cemetery as often as I did in the early days. Perhaps this is because I feel more of Tom's presence around me rather than needing to go to his grave, or more that I am further along in my grief now and my life has grown around it.

Earlier this year I paid a visit to a natural burial ground. I had driven by many times en route to visiting a friend and my curiosity was piqued. What I found was the most peaceful of places, and I have to admit to wondering whether, had I known about it at the time, I would have chosen for Tom to be buried there. Because nature and being outdoors had been such a healing part of my grief, the natural burial ground resonated deeply within me. I have considered planting a tree there in remembrance, and perhaps one day I will get round to doing it. It seemed such a fitting place to remember Tom rather than the rigidity of the cemetery and one that in spite of not being able to visit regularly, would be a wonderful place to go and spend some time.

Professional Perspective

For most people the idea of planning a funeral for your child is simply unbearable. Yet families do this—often in a short period of time, with a huge amount of thought and attention to detail, invariably creating a way of saying goodbye that is both meaningful and memorable. This speaks both of the resilience of parents in crisis and also the skills of those whose job it is to support and guide people at this time. Funeral directors, registrars, spiritual leaders, and hospice and hospital bereavement teams are experienced in guiding families through what needs to be done. Do not feel that you have to do this by yourself, but use the expertise of the professionals around you.

Some families live with the knowledge that their child's life is limited and make plans in advance; others simply have to deal with it at the time. At whatever point you do this, there are some basic decisions to be made: do you want a funeral service that is religious or non-religious? Would you like all of it or any part of it to be private? Is it to be a celebration of the life your child has had or a more sombre goodbye? Do you want to have your child buried or cremated?

Probably the first practicality to think about is registering the death. In England this has to happen within five days of the death and it is best if this is done at a registry office in the area in which the death has occurred. Helen and Douglas House draws families from Oxfordshire and its surrounding counties, but when a child or young adult dies at the hospice the death is registered in Oxford regardless of where the family home is situated. In most places you have to make an appointment with the registrar and you are required to take a medical certificate of the cause of death, which has been signed by a doctor. If you have them available you can also take a birth certificate or NHS medical card, but this is not necessary. The appointment should not take more than thirty minutes and you will be asked for your son's or daughter's full name, date and place of birth, current address, and details of any benefits they had been receiving. The registrar will give you a certificate for burial or cremation ('green form') and a certificate of registration of death. You will have to pay for the death certificate. If there is a post-mortem the coroner will issue any documents as quickly as possible afterwards.

When I first began accompanying families to the registrar's office, I went with the expectation of an emotionally charged appointment, but I could not have been more wrong on that. The registrars manage to find just the right balance of sensitivity and professionalism and enable parents to complete the process with dignity and leave with the paperwork they need and a clear understanding of those details for which it would be required.

The funeral director will need the 'green form' to make firm plans for the funeral. Most people will have little if any previous knowledge of funeral directors, so you might want to ask around in your community for recommendations. Most will not charge for a child's funeral, but there will be fees that they need to pay, for example to the crematorium, which they will pass on to you. Do talk with them about costs and how you will pay for expenses such as the coffin or flowers, which the undertaker will not cover. Janet's son came to Helen and Douglas House on a regular basis and part of her thinking about and planning for his death involved talking with a local funeral director ahead of time about what they could afford. This then was one less thing for her to worry about as the end of her son's life approached. Not everyone has the opportunity or indeed the desire to have these conversations in advance, but it is better to address them as you plan, whenever that is, rather than be shocked by the cost after the event.

You may feel overwhelmed by the number of choices you have to make, from the type of coffin to the music for the service. Take it step by step, and if there are aspects of it that you can delegate, do that. You may have a friend or family member who is great with flowers or very knowledgeable about music, so use their expertise. There will, however, be choices that you probably will not want to delegate.

Coffins come in a surprising array of styles and designs. You will have a choice not only of wood, painted or varnished, but also of materials such as willow or cardboard. You will also have the option of customized decoration. Flowers may be woven into and around willow coffins, and wooden and cardboard coffins can be painted. Helen and Douglas House has seen children and young people buried or cremated in some very creative ways. One Helen and Douglas House guest loved Dr Who, and his coffin was a replica Tardis. Another family chose a white coffin, decorated with pink princesses, reflecting both their daughter's favourite colour and the role she had in the family. Colour themes can be carried through to the clothing which people are invited to wear to the service and even to the funeral cars. Yet another family arranged for a pink hearse to bring their teenage daughter to her humanist service at the crematorium.

You may also want to think about clothes for your son or daughter to wear in the coffin and about anything else you would like placed in beside him or her. Sometimes parents put in a favourite toy or a blanket their child would not be separated from, or perhaps a football jersey or scarf. Parents and siblings may choose to write notes or cards and enclose those also. Helen and Douglas House, like many hospices for children and young adults, has a cooled bedroom in which the young person can be looked after in the days following the death. Families make this space their own, and sometimes parents will choose to dress their son or daughter or to assist hospice staff to do so, in preparation for the funeral. Some parents have chosen to place their child in the coffin, but for many that is a step too far. Allow yourself to do what is right for you. There are no shoulds or oughts in this situation. Each family member has a different point at which they want to say goodbye and that should be respected. A number of parents have talked about their child changing during the time spent in the cooled bedroom, describing the difference as being that the child they now see is no longer the child who was. It is usually at this point that they choose to spend less time with them or to say a final goodbye. You may reach that point sooner or later than other family members, which is fine. However, do not try to impose your choice on others.

If you want a religious service then you may already have connections to a religious community and know who you want to lead the service and how you might like it to be. Many children's hospices and some hospitals will have a chaplaincy or spiritual care team who can be a resource for you. Your funeral director may also be able to help you find the right person to lead the service, whether religious or not. Whatever the nature of the service, you may have to think about music and readings and you may want to consider incorporating some of your son's or daughter's favourite music, poetry, or even stories.

At Helen and Douglas House there are folders of songs and readings which parents can consult for ideas. We also keep a file of orders of service, which again could signpost parents towards what they might like for their own service. Your funeral director can probably help with having an order of service printed, if you decide to have one. Alternatively if you or anyone in your family has the necessary IT skills, this is something you can do for yourself.

Think about who, if anyone, you would like to speak at the service. Perhaps you might like to write something yourself and share it on the day. Family members can be uncertain as to whether they will be able to stand up and speak at the service. Frequently they are surprised by how much they are able to do, but you can relieve some of that anxiety by having on stand-by someone who can step in for you and read what you have prepared. In Chapter 3, I gave the example of a sibling who rehearsed a song for her brother's funeral but also made a recording of it which could be played if she became too emotional or just did not feel able to do it. There is no reason why adults should not have a similar fall-back plan.

The issue of siblings attending the funeral is also covered in Chapter 3. Without major repetition here, the important points are to give children choices, to prepare them for what they will see and experience, and, if they do attend, to ensure that there is a designated adult, other than yourself, who will look after them. If they are too young or choose not to take part in the service, burial, or cremation, it would be good to think about helping them to find an alternative way of saying goodbye.

In addition to choosing words and music, some parents like to have visual images of their child at the funeral. One Helen and Douglas House family made a photo board, which they displayed during the service and which was taken to the tea they held afterwards. They later put it up in what had been Leo's room. Other families have put together a slide show or photo loop, which runs while people are gathering or as they are leaving. You need to check on equipment and how feasible it will be to use it in the place where you will be having the funeral. I would strongly encourage you to delegate this kind of activity to someone else, preferably someone who is familiar with whatever technology you require. You will want to be focused on your child and the service, not distracted by other tasks.

You may want mourners to share some of their memories of your child and you can do this by having available at the funeral a memory book in which people can write. Mark and Lorraine, whose only son died shortly before Christmas, passed out bauble-shaped cards on ribbon and asked that everyone wrote something about Tim on the card. They then took these home and tied them on their Christmas tree.

The decision about burial or cremation will be determined perhaps by religious beliefs, family traditions, and also the life you imagine for yourself. If, for example, you have a family plot at the cemetery, then perhaps there is no decision to be made. I can think of numerous families for whom a child's grave becomes the focus of their grief and a place where they feel connected to the child. Regular visits to the grave, especially early on, are comforting, but may also become restricting. Tanya was reluctant to take a family holiday after her daughter's death, as she hated the idea of leaving her behind at the cemetery. She was also concerned about who would care for the grave. We talked through a plan that saw her pass responsibility for this to family and friends. They agreed to visit the grave while Tanya was gone and to ensure that it was kept neat and tidy as Tanya liked it to be. If it can be hard to leave a grave to go on holiday it will be harder still if you have to move from the area altogether. Sometimes this is one of the reasons families choose cremation. Heather and Simon knew that their work would mean frequent moves so it made no sense to them to bury their daughter in a place they would only live short-term. Cremation was a practical choice for them. Rob and Anya did not need to move on a permanent basis, but travelled a lot and would take their son's ashes with them. Both the need to stay close to the grave and to keep ashes with you will change over time, becoming less compelling, but that sense of connection can influence the decision you make about burial or cremation.

You may want to invite people back after the service. This can take many forms, and I have known parents who have arranged tea and sandwiches or a sit-down meal or have asked everyone to congregate at the local pub. Again there is no right or wrong here. You should do what you feel you can manage emotionally and financially. This is definitely a responsibility that can be delegated! Family members and friends will be only too happy to be useful and to take on the very practical task of finding a venue or making lots of tea and cakes. Think, too, about pacing yourself. This will be an exhausting day.

Tracy talked about taking breaks during Tom's reception. Other parents have arranged a gathering and spent a short time there, leaving family and friends to carry on eating and talking.

'I just don't know if I can do it' is the most frequently voiced fear about the funeral. As with the visits to the registrar's office I have been consistently awed and impressed by the resilience parents demonstrate in seeing through their son's or daughter's funeral. Of course, it is emotional and exhausting, but every parent who has voiced that concern has a found a way through.

Separate from, but related to the decision about burial or cremation, are thoughts about a headstone. At first this may appear straightforward, but what I have seen with families is that this is a choice laden with meaning and one not made easily. It comes up in individual visits with families and also in parent support groups. One group in fact elected to spend an entire session thinking about and sharing their experiences of choosing a headstone. I think that some of the difficulty stems from the erection of the headstone having a very final feel to it. Some parents feel the weight of it being the last thing they can do for their son or daughter. Further, while it may not be the last word on your child's life it will be the enduring word, and parents simply feel the pressure to have it right.

Once again you will be faced with a number of choices and decisions regarding the type of stone you use, the size and shape of the headstone, and the wording. Make sure that you or your stonemason are very clear about the cemetery regulations. I worked with a family who, shortly after their daughter's headstone was erected, received a letter saying that it would have to be removed. Apparently it did not comply with the cemetery's regulations. The family successfully challenged this and the headstone remains there, but you will save yourself considerable heartache and distress if you check all of this out in advance.

The most difficult decision seems to be about the wording for the stone. The best advice to offer here is that you should take the time you need to word it the way you want. Some families feel that there is an element of neglect about not having a headstone in place quickly enough and parents often feel pressure to have it put in place by the first anniversary. You can, though, take as long as you need.

Headstones are expensive, and once the wording is literally set in stone there will be little option to change it, so take your time. You and your partner or family will reach a point where you can agree about what looks and feels right, or come to a compromise with which you can live.

As I said at the beginning of this chapter, parents somehow manage to do the unthinkable and to create a funeral for their child that is meaningful and memorable. Sometimes the thinking, planning, and taking pride in arranging it the way they want it is what helps families through those first few days.

Things to Remember

- Be guided by the professionals. Funeral directors, registrars etc. do this all day, every day and have expertise to share
- Talk about costs and be realistic about what you can afford
- Think about what you regard as important to include in the service; paying attention to what feels right to share and what you want to be private
- Check out cemetery regulations regarding headstones and don't feel pressured to put one up until you are ready
- Accept all offers of help
- Delegate what you can!

Your Notes

Chapter 10

Creating and retaining memories

Parent's Perspective

Over the years since Tom died I have made many attempts to create memories, both tangible things and more private ones in my own head. Many, many hours have been spent lost in my memories, and at first I found it so painful it would reduce me to tears.

The music that I chose to have played at his funeral was actually playing on our iPod dock at the moment he died. That song (which happens to be on one of my favourite albums) will forever have a bittersweet memory for me now. In the first months following Tom's death, I liked to listen to that song, along with the rest of the album, and I would find some comfort from it, but I remember friends saying that they wouldn't be able to listen to it anymore. As time has passed, I don't play the album quite so much, but when I hear the song played randomly I just let the memory fill my head and wonder why it is that I don't play it as much as I used to. I have many songs and pieces of music that all have connections and memories to Tom and the things we used to do together. There is nothing I like to do more than sit down and put my iPod on shuffle and see what happens . . . what will play and where it will take me. I find music particularly healing and relaxing. It is my choice of escapism every time.

I have many, many photographs of Tom, and of Charlie, and again, in a serendipitous moment when browsing through someone else's Sunday supplement, I happened to find an article about Bob Books. At the time, I never knew that you could do such a thing as produce your own book—professionally printed!—rather than just the traditional photo album. My interest was immediately piqued and I set about downloading the software, which was free. I decided to make a book for Charlie as a Christmas present for the first Christmas without Tom (Fig. 10.1). I wanted to find a picture of them together for every year since Charlie had been born. It took what felt like months trawling through all my photos making my final selection. I then used the software to upload them and added some dates to make it relevant. The hardest part was choosing the design elements given that the choice was huge! Tom's favourite book ever was *The Very Hungry Caterpillar*, and so on the last page I used the opening line. I also used the quote 'It takes two boys to make one brother' which I thought was perfect for the first page.

I called the book *Remembering Tom* and I gave it to Charlie in a private moment on Christmas morning. I like the fact that I have often had to put it back on the bookshelf in Charlie's room, as to me that is a sign that it has been looked at often. When I help out with the bereavement training sessions at St Mary's Hospital I always take the book with me as I like to show it to the doctors there to illustrate who I am talking about. I have also shared it at my bereaved parents group and at other workshops and training sessions. Charlie has always allowed me to use it and I hope that he is proud of his contribution.

Photographs are, of course, the most obvious way of saving visual memories to spend time with later, and since Tom died I have spent more time taking photographs and I do regret not taking photos of the tinier details of him for me study rather than the bigger picture of perhaps him with other people. I have noticed that over the last few years I have become quite obsessed with macro photography as I talked about in Chapter 2, where I get really close to my subject and focus on the finer details. Oh, how I wish I had a macro lens to capture Tom. It is these tiny details of him that I miss dreadfully—the things that perhaps I took for granted before. I have a few videos of Tom that were taken on occasions while we were on holiday, but I have only ever watched one of them once since he died. I am not really sure why this is, as I know other parents have taken much comfort from watching videos of their children. Perhaps it is because I never really took many videos and so they are not part of my memory storing strategy.

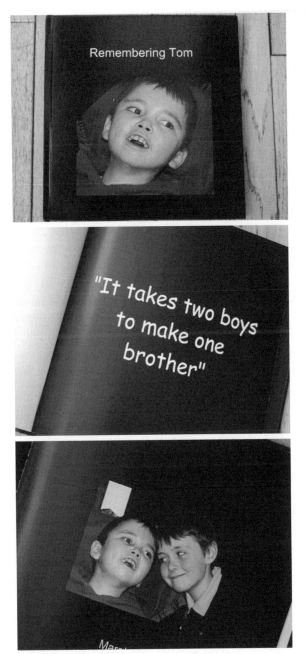

Fig. 10.1 *Remembering Tom*: a book for Charlie.

I have mentioned in other chapters throughout the book that I regularly blog and I have found this is a wonderful way to create and store memories. My blog is not about any one thing in particular, more of an online journal where I can record bits and pieces of my life in general and share it with others. When I first started writing it I didn't talk about Tom, but as time passed I felt the need to share this most important part of my life. Since sharing, I have sometimes written about my memories of Tom and I always mark his anniversary and birthday on my blog. I have used it as a space to capture things that I want to remember and often wonder if (had I known such a thing existed!) I would have perhaps chosen to blog about our family life while Tom was still alive. A post that springs to mind is one where I shared snapshots of places around the house where I could find reminders of Tom's presence. I took photos of the funny dinosaur shower-head in his bathroom and the collection of Beanie Babies above his bed—little things of his that I wanted to record forever.

I have always found writing to be very cathartic. When Tom first became ill and was admitted to The Children's Trust for his rehabilitation I started writing a diary for him on a monthly basis that I would send out to family and friends so that they could keep track of his progress. Looking back, I can recognize this as one of the first coping skills I developed to handle difficult situations during what was a very stressful time. My days were busy, tiring, and completely turned on their head in those early days of Tom's initial illness when he was four and I had Charlie, who was just a year old, to care for too and so posting out an update regularly seemed a good idea to keep in touch with everyone when I really did not have time to physically see or even speak to them. I carried on writing Tom's diary for eight years and over that period of time I was soon circulating it to more than sixty people all over the world. I was often praised for having the discipline to write so regularly but I can honestly say that I never found it a chore. I was always very strict with myself about the length of the diary (two sides of A4, maximum) and as the months were always so busy with the normal routines of our life it was never difficult to fill those pages. As my skills on the computer improved over the years, I learnt how to include photos which were always a good filler if I found myself short on words. I now have several files of written memories that I absolutely treasure. I stopped writing the diary in October 2005 when I had the more realistic prognosis for Tom. For some reason, I was unable to write anymore. I had always written the diary in the first person, as though Tom was telling everybody what he had been doing, and I just found that I could not continue in that vein any longer.

I still like to keep a journal intermittently and writing thoughts down is a very healing way to help process them. I tend not to write a diary as such and seem to find more unusual ways to keep track of things and store my memories. I have found ideas in the online communities about keeping a journal and have found short-term projects to be a creative way of preserving my thoughts and ideas. Although they are not necessarily focused on grief or bereavement, I do often find that these subjects permeate my writing. At the moment, I am taking part in a *52 in 52* weekly journal of lists. The lists can consist of hopes for the future or things from the past. I choose not to share mine online but I find it a useful tool for making me think about my life now and how it is shaping up without Tom in it.

On my travels around the Internet over the last few years I have been interested to see that in the USA it has become popular to make a keepsake quilt to remember a loved one, using clothes or other significant fabrics. I think this is a wonderful idea and something that I would, one day, like to do. As I write, Tom's wardrobe and drawers are exactly as they were in April 2006 and I would really like to think that sometime I will be able to have something made from his clothes rather than get rid of them. I am guessing that it will not happen until I choose to move from this house as I have no urge to change things in his bedroom at the present time. In the early days of my grief, I would often just go and sit in his wardrobe and allow myself to be surrounded by his clothes. Nowadays, I sometimes go in there and open it up and find a sense of melancholy fills me with a gentle sadness about the passing of time.

The task of changing things around the house is a very difficult one, as there are deep-rooted memories connected with possessions and the space that they are in. My house was designed specifically for Tom after his brain injury to accommodate his necessary hoists and lift. He had a room downstairs that was the hub of our home. It was used for all his daily activities and had some multi-sensory equipment in there too. As Charlie grew into a teenager, we decided to use the space downstairs and so I moved my study/workroom into Tom's multi-sensory room and we made a den for Charlie in what was my study/workroom. I now love spending time in this room again and am filled with many happy memories while I go about my day and it has, once more, become the hub of my home. I find an innate sense of peace and inspiration when I am working in there.

In pride of place on the bookshelf in my workroom is a box containing all the cards and letters of condolence I received after Tom died. They are a very precious reminder of the way Tom was loved by all who knew him, and the words that are written there illustrate the huge legacy left by one who was so young. They are among my most treasured possessions and I have found myself immersed in them on many occasions.

Professional Perspective

One of the anxieties you may experience early in your grief is the fear of forgetting; therefore finding ways of creating and retaining memories takes on a significance of its own. It is important not just to bereaved parents but equally so to those who know their son or daughter's life will be limited. At one of our workshops for parents in this latter group we asked them for suggestions of interesting topics that would be useful to them for future sessions. Along with requests for self-care and managing stress parents also asked for a workshop on creating memories. The knowledge that their child's life would be short inspired them to want to think about ways of recording it. Not every parent can so clearly anticipate life after their son or daughter has died, so on the day of the workshop it was a small group but there were still useful ideas discussed. We tapped into Tracy's creative expertise and she shared the many ways in which she had woven Tom and memories of him into an on-going family life.

Tracy has written about how she has gone about retaining memories and we will also look at how other families have managed it. Please think of these simply as ideas and suggestions, definitely not as a 'to do' list. Even in families who do not have the added responsibility of providing constant care for a sick child, parents typically find it hard to make time for organizing photographs or recording the big moments, so do not feel bad if you do not have everything neatly logged. And for bereaved parents many months may pass before you feel able to look at photographs or reflect on some of the fabulous times with your child without it causing searing pain.

When I began supporting Tracy she showed me the beautiful diary she had kept during the years since Tom's brain injury. It is a work of art and I remember being astonished at how she had found the time to do it and to continue to do it for so long. As I talked to Tracy about it, though, I came to understand that it served many purposes, and although it took time, it also saved Tracy time. Initially she wrote it as a way of keeping people informed. In sending out regular bulletins she did not have to respond to lots of individual phone calls or emails, and when you are caring for someone round the clock that time is precious. As she wrote it in Tom's voice it put him at the centre and gave their supporters an insight into what life was like for him.

And while it was not her original intention, the writing became therapeutic for Tracy. Since Tom died it has become a treasured record of a significant part of both his and the family's life that they can return to time and time again.

Not everyone will have the hours, inclination, or perseverance for that kind of activity, so do not feel bad if you cannot imagine writing this kind of diary, or in fact any other kind of journal. You will have your own memories to access at whatever point it becomes important to you, or you find you have the energy to try to order or record them.

One of the first times when you may feel motivated to do this is the funeral. We talked in Chapter 9 about families preparing photo boards or slide shows for that occasion, and in either writing your own personal tribute to your son or daughter or asking someone else to do it you will be tapping into your memories. As also mentioned in that chapter, the funeral can be an opportunity to ask people attending to write down a short memory which they would like to share with you, and then you will have that to keep.

As time goes by you may find friends and family offering you their own mementoes in assorted shapes and forms. These may be cards or letters previously sent by your child—perhaps something they have made, or photographs or home movies. For one family a close friend made a DVD of every snippet she had on film and gave it to them. This was a wonderful gift, not just because of the cherished images, but also because of the thoughtfulness and care it demonstrated. Another family was sent a booklet of photographs from their daughter's school, some of which showed her enjoying things about which they had not previously heard. Not everyone around you will think to do this for you. In fact some people will worry about upsetting you with these reminders, so, when you are ready, do not be afraid to ask people to share whatever they have stored away, whether in their head or in a photograph album.

These memories will be important to more than you, the parents. One Helen and Douglas House family gathered all of the film they had of their son and had it professionally edited and made into a DVD. They then bought enough copies of it to give to grandparents and aunts and uncles, ensuring that they each had their own personal collection of memories. In putting the DVD together these parents were thinking not just about themselves and the extended family, they knew that they were planning to have more children and part of their thinking at the time was that this would be another way in which their future children would get to know their older brother. These children are still young, but the DVD will be there for them whenever the time is right.

However you gather and store memories, think about how you want them to be used. Is it something that you will want only for yourself or will you want to show it to other people? If you do, remember that DVDs can be lost or damaged, as can photographs, whether stored in an album or on your computer. Make sure that any of the recorded memories you cannot live without are backed up or that you have them in duplicate. If you have photo booklets or you write a life story book, again think about a second copy. If you only have one copy, then perhaps laminating it will help to preserve it, especially if you are making this for a child to look at.

You will probably want to hold on to more than images and sounds. Some families take hand or footprints when the child dies and often a lock of hair. You may have a special box or container for these, or you may keep them in a larger memory box, alongside other essential items. Many people now are familiar with the idea of a memory box, and putting one together is something you can do individually or as a family. As we discussed in Chapter 3, you may want to include things that stimulate the different senses. As well as photographs or a ticket from a special event you might put in an item of clothing or a favourite belonging of your son or daughter. Whether the smell you associate with your child was baby lotion or Lynx shower gel, think about capturing some of that in the box, too. Do not underestimate the memory-evoking power of different scents. I have supported so many mothers who have talked about their inability to wash their child's bedding or sweater and who have found it comforting to be able to inhale some of their son or daughter's unique smell. You can buy, or make, and decorate your own memory box and, of course, it need not be a box. You can choose any kind of container that works for you. Alongside the box or instead of one you might want to make a memory book or write a life story, again with contributions from people who were part of your child's life.

There can be friction in families about the appropriateness of holding onto your son or daughter's belongings or disagreement about the speed with which they are removed or hidden. The consistent message throughout this book is that there is no fixed time line or order in which you should do things. I know parents who have wanted grandparents or friends to remove all their child's medical equipment and supplies from the house before they return to it. In the case of a baby death it was the crib that had to be taken away. In contrast, other families were desolate when the day finally came that another child needed that special piece of equipment, which they had on loan, and it was removed from the home. There will be some of your child's belongings which you may never want to be parted from and others that you will let go of gradually. As with so many things it is a question of balance. What does it matter if your son's or daughter's jacket still hangs by the door because you like having it there to see and touch as you go in and out? Does it become a problem though if his or her room is maintained as a shrine, which no one is allowed to enter or touch? If you have lots of photographs on display do they represent the whole family—siblings as well as the child who has died? If not, what does that communicate to your living children? The goal is to capture and retain memories which you can integrate into your life, rather than have your life dominated by the preservation of a room or particular belongings.

Tracy has referred to the idea of using favourite items of clothing to make a keepsake quilt. By doing this, or something similar, the clothes will no longer be tucked away, but will become a cherished part of family life. If you feel you do not have the creative skills for this but would like to do something similar think about whoever you have in your family or circle of friends who might enjoy taking on a project like this for you.

When Tracy was in one of the parent groups she brought along the book which she described for you and which she had made and printed for Charlie. I know other parents then did this for themselves. There are several websites which offer this service and the books can be kept just for you or given as gifts to other family members. Again if you like this idea, but would not know where to begin, ask for help from the family and friends who are there for you and have the skills for this.

In the early stages of grief parents can feel overwhelmed by difficult memories. You may also interpret memories differently; something which is painful to you may be comforting to your partner, and vice versa. Parents do usually report, however, that this changes over time and as well as there being less focus on the painful memories they are able to think about the good days, too. We have concentrated on structured and organized ways of retaining memories, but not all of us work that way and neither do memories themselves. They can be tied to a place or piece of music or a scent, which you might just about capture in a box, but you will probably also bump up against them when you are not expecting to do so. Memories cannot all be corralled into a safe space.

What is more important than the way in which you keep memories is that you can access them and share them. Helen and Douglas House holds annual remembrance days for all of the families whose children and young adults have used the hospice. Parents come to remember their son or daughter, but they also come because it is a place where they can share memories. Families are keen to talk with staff who looked after their children, but also to reminisce with other parents about their time at the hospice. There is no need for memory boxes or photo books, as the place and relationships are rich with recollections.

As part of the closing session of some of our parents' groups, we would invite participants to bring a significant item belonging to their son or daughter, and if they wanted to, to talk about it in the group. It made no difference whether they had made boxes or books or if reminders and belongings were scattered randomly through their house, each parent came with a toy or a sweater or whatever, and talked about why it was meaningful. There were tears, but also much laughter as parents relished the chance to tell their stories and talk about their child. And surely that is the real way we keep memories alive—talking about them and sharing. By all means make a box or book or a quilt of memories, but resist the urge to keep them tucked away. Share them and the other memories in your head with the people around you. Use the memories to make your son or daughter a part of everyday conversation and, in that way, you will maintain the bond that you have with him or her and keep the memories alive.

Things to Remember

Store memories in a way that makes sense for you. You might consider:

- Journals
- Photo albums
- Photo books
- Music compilations
- DVDS
- Keepsake quilt
- Memory boxes

Make sure you have back ups, if it is possible to do that. Gather other people's memories to add to your own and talk about your memories and share your recollections

Your Notes

Chapter 11

Facing the future

Parent's Perspective

The question I ask myself on an almost daily basis is 'Who am I now?'. When Tom died I just could not imagine how I would continue living my life without him as part of it. I could not imagine how I would find the inclination or inspiration to do anything other than the most fundamental of tasks. I could not imagine how I would ever be able to feel anything other than totally devastated.

It has been a revelation to me in the process of writing this book with Christine that I can recognize each of the stages of grief that she describes without having been aware of them at the time. I find it a huge comfort (and relief) that the way I felt was pretty much, dare I say, normal.

Making the decision early on in my grief that I would not try to 'get over it' has been the keystone to the way I now feel able to face the future. I have been guided along the way with support from bereaved parents, the courage I have seen in Charlie, the memory of Tom, and, of course, gentle guidance from Christine herself. I have applied the same tactics to handling my grief as I did when Tom was alive, namely having an open mind and trusting my gut instinct. It has been immeasurably helpful to see in diagrammatic form the way the stages of grief have been identified by researchers in the field, particularly the dual process model that Christine described in Chapter 1. I am a classic visual learner, and when I see something presented in such a way it really helps my understanding. My bereavement has been the biggest lesson of my life.

I have come to realize that just because I choose not to visit Tom's grave regularly or cry a lot, it does not mean that I am not grieving in the way that is expected of me. I am grieving the way I grieve. I have learnt to have faith in doing things in my own way and in my own time. I can admit to making mistakes and bad decisions, but feel I have learnt from them so that they are not perceived by me to be necessarily negative experiences. I have found things from unexpected sources that have resonated deeply with me and which I have remembered at crucial times or put into practice where necessary.

When I have had a harsh opinion of myself, I found comfort from a book called *Buddhism for mothers with lingering questions*.[1] It is not a book about bereavement or grief, but a book about raising children. As I wrote in Chapter 7, I am not a particularly religious person but I found the Buddhist teachings discussed in that book especially helpful in remembering how I chose to parent Tom and how I continue to parent Charlie. I was encouraged to read that it was healthy to try to stay true to myself—rather than doing what I felt perhaps others expected of me, I did what felt instinctively right for me. I read the words in that book and felt as though they were unravelling some of the jumble of thoughts and emotions that filled my head. The book also introduced me to the concept of mindfulness. Knowing about mindfulness allowed me to give myself permission to accept the way I was feeling at the present moment, acknowledge it, and, if it was a negative experience, know that it, like bad weather, would pass. This may sound a little like I am belittling the extent of my grief, but I believe that it goes to show how much it has changed over time and that I can recognize that my life has grown around it to such an extent that I can see it in my mind's eye exactly as illustrated in Tonkin's diagram in Chapter 2.

When I started to read Klass's *The Spiritual Lives of Bereaved Parents*[2] I was fascinated to learn of the references to Eastern traditions alongside those of the Western ones I was to an extent familiar with. I found that by taking a holistic view of my circumstances once again, I could somehow make sense of them. I was relieved to read that as a bereaved parent I found myself in the recognized state of being in unchartered territory, whether it be religious or otherwise. I was comforted to read about the idea of 'continuing bonds'. It seemed to cement the feelings that had surfaced within me that my grief was most definitely not something that I was going to get over. It clarified the fact that I wanted Tom to be an important part of my life forever, not just a memory. He remains my inspiration and driving force to do all the things, whether they be big or small, that I do on a daily basis. I am reminded of him each time I do things with Charlie—that they are and always will be brothers.

One of the other recognized elements of continuing bonds in those who are *well along in their grief* is the decision to share your experience to support others who have been bereaved. I was honoured to have been asked by the family support team at Helen and Douglas House to come to an interview with the prospect of training to do peer-to-peer support at the hospice. In spite of being less bereaved than the usual criteria required, I was accepted onto the programme and have been supporting other bereaved parents since my training was completed in 2010. I have found it an enormous privilege to be able to sit and listen to my peers in a one-to-one setting and provide a non-judgmental ear and empathy for what they have shared with me.

Likewise, when I was asked if I would consider taking part in a bereavement training programme that was being offered to paediatric registrars in London facilitated by The Child Bereavement Charity, I was more than happy to talk with them of my experiences as a bereaved parent on the understanding that it would serve to help others. The responses I have received from these sessions have been amazing and I have taken it as a huge compliment to have been allowed to be as passionate about the death of my child as I was about his life.

In Chapter 1 I also talked about my need to be outside. I have learnt that being outdoors and taking particular notice of nature and the natural world has had a therapeutic effect on me that is recognized, as Christine has talked about in Chapter 1. I have often felt stifled when indoors and have struggled to motivate myself into doing anything at all. On these occasions I have taken my camera outdoors and captured what I have seen. This, in turn, seems to have been the motivating force to then actually *do* something positive and creative. As a consequence, I now have thousands of photographs that are filed on my computer that give me enormous pleasure to look at. I have joined photo sharing communities and this in turn has helped me to find a place in which to feel comfortable.

The creative energy that I found in making a life for Tom and Charlie after Tom's initial illness surfaced again after Tom died, and although it took a while I discovered ways that I could channel it into doing something productive. I rediscovered hobbies and interests that had been long forgotten, and with the help of the online community that I then found myself joining, I began to teach myself new ways to pursue my creativity. Initially, they did not require huge amounts of energy, which was exactly what I needed at the time as I simply did not have that. They were gentle introductions into filling the time which I found myself to have in copious amounts.

I have found the confidence to teach others what I have learnt and have been able to encourage small circles of like-minded people to want to get together on a regular basis to craft and to find inspiration from each other. I am a firm believer that creativity promotes healing, and this has been communicated to me from some of the women in my craft group who have had serious illnesses. It has become important to me to make my life meaningful, and if by teaching someone to make something, a cushion perhaps, which in turn gives them a sense of achievement then I am satisfied that my philosophy of sharing is being put to good use. I have started to feel comfortable in acknowledging my continued relationship with Tom in this newfound community and do not feel afraid to comment that if my sewing machine starts doing its own thing (which it does on a regular basis!) it is just Tom playing about.

I do not feel that my grief is *resolved as much as it will be* at this present time, rather that I am *well along in my grief.* However, I do agree with a comment by another bereaved mother (who was in the former category) in that my grief now is gentler and that it is about aching in gentler ways. I am committed to maintaining my continuing bonds with Tom and fully recognize the importance of ritual and customs that have come about since him dying. I find myself happy to continue going to remembrance services, whether they be at the hospital where he was treated or at the hospice, because I enjoy giving myself an allocated time to simply remember without any other distractions. Having said that, when circumstances have prevented me from attending, I have tried not to worry about missing such an event.

A noticeable change that I have begun to recognize is one where I find myself beginning to make plans and allow ideas to formulate about my future beyond the next few days or week. This is something new to me, and makes me realize how far I have come and how much my grief has changed over time. My perception of time has started to become less frightening in spite of knowing that Charlie is growing up fast and that he will soon want to spread his wings, which will leave me with an empty nest.

This feels like a giant step forward from the twenty-minute time-span that I talked about in Chapter 1. Back in those early days, twenty minutes was barely tolerable but, without me really being aware of it, those units of time gradually became more manageable; eventually I was able to add them together until whole days were filled with activities or even boring domestic chores.

Professional Perspective

I suspect that some of you reading this will hate the idea of a chapter about the future. When grief is raw, we want to go back to the past; the present feels unbearable and the future is completely unimaginable. The prospect of years stretching ahead, bereft of that special person, can feel like a life sentence. It is hard to imagine a time when you might enjoy or look forward to something. But the truth is that by far the majority of bereaved parents do gradually come to that place. They find themselves doing, thinking, and feeling things which previously were inconceivable.

Reflect on some of what Tracy has written. In Chapter 1 she described days spent sitting on the sofa, her struggle to come to terms with the lack of structure which Tom's care had necessitated, and the jumble of thoughts and feelings which she was experiencing. Look at how this contrasts with her life now. She is engaged with the world, yet still holds a place for Tom within it. This is not just Tracy's experience; it is also that of most of the parents with whom I have worked. They do slowly re-build or re-create a life that still holds their son or daughter, but also one in which they experience hope and joy.

How do parents do it? There is no magic potion and it is, of course, different for everyone, but there are some common factors involved. One is the passage of time. Parents are frequently offended by people telling them that time heals—to them it seems that the opposite is true. The more days and months that go by, the longer it is since they have held, seen, or touched their son or daughter and they yearn for that. I also question whether time alone heals, but have clearly seen that feelings *do* change with time. They become less raw and less random. Some parents have described this as being like a changing pattern of waves. In the first months after being bereaved, parents describe being hit by tsunami after tsunami of painful feelings, in the wake of which they barely get back on their feet before the next one strikes. However, they notice that over time the waves lose some of their strength and that there is longer between each onslaught, allowing increasing time for parents to get their breath back. Little-by-little they record the waves of emotion losing some of their frequency and intensity (Fig. 11.1).

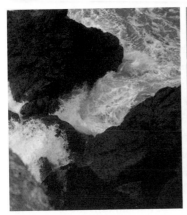 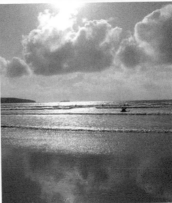

Fig. 11.1 Wave patterns.

As the wave pattern slows and becomes less fierce, it allows energy to return, which makes it more likely that you can begin to re-engage with life. Instead of going through the motions at work or in parenting your other children, you will slowly but surely find yourself becoming more present and available. It is not only about the passage of time, though. You may have to consciously choose to permit yourself not just to re-engage but to allow yourself some enjoyment in the process.

Sometimes others may prod or encourage you to do this. I remember working with Ella, an adult sibling whose sister had died three years previously. Ella's parents were about to go on holiday and it was obvious to Ella that although her mother was excited and looking forward to it, she felt she should not be. Her mother, therefore, behaved as if she were doing something she would prefer not to do and this influenced how other family members felt they could anticipate the break. Ella gently challenged her mother and suggested that she was still allowed to have a life and to enjoy it, and Ella was right in thinking and saying that. Pleasure or happiness in your life does not constitute a betrayal of your son or daughter who has died. Neither does it mean that you are forgetting him or her. Strange as it may seem, you can acknowledge the loss and at the same time be happy about other aspects of your life.

It is not simply that feelings will change over time, but you have a choice to make about whether you allow yourself to accept the change and give yourself permission to feel the good, the bad, and everything in between.

Parents often express concern that if they let go of their pain they will lose their son or daughter again. It can feel as if the pain is what anchors you together, but the continuing bond between you does not have to one of pain. Dennis Klass[3] quotes from a mother whose son died five years previously, describing her decision to let go of her pain and allow herself happiness. Like most parents she was afraid of forgetting her son, but recognized that she had become accustomed to her pain and even drew comfort from it. Ultimately she realized that her son's life was about more than pain—it was also about joy and living. She found that when she let go of the pain, she made room for happiness and that far from forgetting him, she found her memories remained and that they were comforting.

This is a good point at which to remind ourselves of what Klass has to say about parental grief and its meaning: 'The end of grief is not severing the bond with the dead child, but integrating the child into the parent's life in a different way than when the child was alive.' The parent referred to above illustrates a part of that process. We know that transforming that bond can be a long and painful process, but it is exactly what, with time and effort, parents do. Klass writes about parents themselves observing the changing form of their grief, from the early painful participation in groups to becoming a facilitator, to finding that they no longer needed the groups. This is a progression that I have also seen in families. Some of those parents who, like Tracy, came in trepidation to their first group or workshop, have later become peer supporters or co-facilitators of other parent support programmes, and have recognized that they have moved from a place of need to one of feeling and being able to give. That particular type of transition may not be part of your grief process, but it will happen in other areas of your life. You will not continue to be defined by your sadness and pain. Think back to Chapter 2 and Lois Tonkin's model of growing around grief. Like the mother mentioned above, other parents before you have discovered ways to retain the memory of their son or daughter and to re-build a life that encompasses those memories.

The markers of change will be different for each of you, but there will be small and larger indicators that your grief is subsiding. You may notice the absence of that horrible panicky feeling when you first wake up or realize that you can look at photographs and smile. For one mum her significant change marker was being able to move from the house where she had lived with her son and trust that she would take the sad and the happy memories with her. I have witnessed parents make bold decisions about a promotion or training opportunity, as well as taking smaller steps back into life and reconnecting with others. Give yourself permission to acknowledge these steps and try not to feel that you cannot let go of the pain. Your son or daughter and his or her memories can be with you, independent of pain.

Know, too, that even as your life expands around your grief and there is more space for happiness, you will not be without sadness. Even as the years go by there will still be days and events that will sting. Neither will you be exempt from other losses and difficulties. The death of your child will not protect you or your family from further illnesses, or financial difficulties, or any of the other problems that are part of life. Tracy wrote earlier about feeling almost fearless since Tom died, and I think that for some parents there is a sense of having survived the worst and the accompanying thought that nothing can affect them so powerfully again. Whether that is true or not, you will face future challenges and difficulties armed with what you have learned about yourself since your child's death and the resilience you have developed to survive it.

There is no neat way to tie up this chapter, or indeed this book, for neither grief nor the future lend themselves to tidy packages. In Chapter 1 I encouraged you to borrow from other parents' experiences and from that to know that that there *are* ways through this. Remind yourself again of that and trust that this is not the end of your life. You can have hope for the future. The poem 'I carry your heart with me' by E. E. Cummings (http://www.poetryfoundation.org/poem/179622), which has, from time to time, been part of Helen and Douglas House remembrance services, beautifully illustrates the continuing bond and that sense of carrying your children with you. The lives of bereaved parents do move forward and within those lives parents find ways of taking their son or daughter with them.

References

1. Napthali, S. (2008) *Buddhism for mothers with lingering questions.* Orion, London.
2. Klass, D. (1999) *The spiritual lives of bereaved parents,* 1st edn. Routledge, London.
3. Klass, D. (1996) The deceased child in the psychic and social worlds of bereaved parents during the resolution of grief. In: *Continuing bonds: new understandings of grief* (ed. D. Klass, P.R. Silverman, and S.L. Nickman), pp. 199–216. Taylor and Francis, London.

Your Notes

Resource list

Organizations and Charities

Brake

This road safety charity runs a helpline for anyone bereaved as a result of a road crash. Brake runs free courses to train people to educate young drivers about the consequences of dangerous driving behaviours. Helpline: 0845 603 8570; www.brake.org.uk

Care for the Family

Care for the Family is a national charity which aims to promote strong family life and to help those who face family difficulties. Tel: 029 2081 0800; www.careforthefamily.org.uk

The Child Bereavement Charity

Provides support to families and professionals when a child dies or when a child is bereaved of someone important in their lives. Services offered include a support and information line, Buckinghamshire-based family bereavement support service, interactive website with a families and professionals forum, resources, and professionals training programme. Tel: 01494 446648; www.childbereavement.org.uk

Child Death Helpline

Telephone helpline for anyone affected by the death of a child, from pre-birth to the death of an adult child, however long ago, and whatever the circumstances. It is staffed by experienced and trained bereaved parent volunteers. Freephone helpline: 0800 282986 (Mon–Fri 10 a.m.–1 p.m.; Tue and Wed 1–3 p.m.; every evening 7–10 p.m.); www.childdeathhelpline.org.uk

Childhood Bereavement Network

The Childhood Bereavement Network (CBN) is the hub for those working with bereaved children, young people, and their families across the UK. They underpin their members' work with essential support and representation: bringing them together across localities, disciplines, and sectors to improve bereavement care for children. CBN has a directory of all local child bereavement services, which can be accessed via their website. Tel: 020 7843 6309; www.childhood-bereavementnetwork.org.uk; e-mail: cbn@ncb.org.uk

The Compassionate Friends

An organization of bereaved parents and their families offering understanding, support, and encouragement to others after the death of a child or children. They also offer support, advice, and information to other relatives, friends, and professionals who are helping the family. Tel: 0845 123 2304; www.tcf.org.uk

Cruse Bereavement Care

Cruse is the largest bereavement support organization for both adults and children in the UK. They provide one-to-one support to anyone who has suffered bereavement, together with a telephone helpline. Their website gives further information and contact details for local branches. Tel: 0844 477 9400; www.cruse.org.uk

Cruse Bereavement Care Scotland

Cruse Bereavement Care Scotland provides similar support to Cruse in England, Wales, and Northern Ireland. Tel: 01738 444807; www.crusescotland.org.uk

CRY—Cardiac Risk in the Young

Cardiac Risk in the Young (CRY) supports those bereaved through sudden cardiac death in the young (also known as SADS, SDS), and has a surgery supporters network for young people (aged 14–35) diagnosed with a cardiac condition. CRY promotes heart screening and ECG testing programmes, and funds the CRY Centre for Sports

Cardiology and the CRY Centre for Cardiac Pathology. Tel: 01737 363222; www.c-r-y.org.uk; e-mail: cry@c-r-y.org.uk

Foundation for the Study of Infant Deaths (FSID)

FSID funds research, supports families whose babies have died suddenly and unexpectedly, and gives 'safe sleep' advice. Helpline: 0808 802 6868; www.fsid.org.uk

The Grandparents Association

A national charity which supports all grandparents and their families. Have a helpline and expert advice, whatever the problem. Helpline: 0845 4349585; www.grandparents-association.org.uk; E-mail: info@ grandparents-association.org.uk

Miscarriage Association

Miscarriage can be a very unhappy, frightening, and lonely experience. If you have been affected by miscarriage, ectopic pregnancy, or molar pregnancy, the Miscarriage Association aims to provide the information and support that you need to help you through. Helpline: 01924 200799 (Mon–Fri 9 a.m.–4 p.m.); www.miscarriageassociation. org.uk

SADS UK—Sudden Arrhythmic Death Syndrome

National cardiac charity providing support to families and individuals affected by a sudden unexpected death. Qualified counsellors and support contacts offer assistance after the death of a child or young spouse. Retreats for the bereaved. Also supports those diagnosed with cardiac conditions and donates cardiac equipment to medical establishments. Tel: 01277 811215; www.sadsuk.org; e-mail: info@sadsuk.org

Samaritans

Provides confidential non-judgemental emotional support 24 hours a day to people who are experiencing feelings of distress or despair, including those which could lead to suicide. Tel: 08457 909090; www. samaritans.org; e-mail: jo@samaritans.org

SAMM—Support After Murder and Manslaughter

Supporting those who have been bereaved as a result of murder or manslaughter, through a telephone helpline, information, and other activities, including local groups. Helpline: 0845 8723440; www. samm.org.uk

Sand Rose

Provides a place where bereaved families can start to re-build their lives. It offers a quiet, peaceful haven where families can be independent but know that they are in a suitable environment. The project, which works in collaboration with local and national bereavement organizations, extends to anyone who has experienced bereavement, although there is a particular emphasis on young families. www. sandrose.org.uk

SANDS—Still and Neonatal Death Charity

Offers support when your baby dies during pregnancy or after birth. Helpline: 020 7436 5881; www.uk-sands.org

Survivors of Bereavement by Suicide [previously known as SOBS]

Providing help and support to those bereaved by the suicide of a relative or close friend. They provide information, a helpline, and other activities, including local groups and events throughout the UK. Helpline: 0844 561 6855; www.uk-sobs.org.uk

Together for short lives—ACT and Children's Hospices UK

Provides information to families and professionals involved in palliative care for *children* with life-threatening or terminal conditions; www.togetherforshortlives.org.uk

Winston's Wish

Winston's Wish supports bereaved children and young people up to the age of 18 through a whole range of activities, including a helpline, group work, residential events and resources. Helpline: 08452 030405; www.winstonswish.org.uk

Other resources

Homeopathy

British Homeopathic Association, Hahnemann House, 29 Park Street, WestLuton LU1 3BE. Tel: 01582 408675; www.britishhomeopathic. org; e-mail: info@britishhomeopathic.org

Bob Books

Photographic books, calendars etc. (as described by Tracy in Chapter 10): www.bobbooks.co.uk

Further reading

Aldridge, J. (2007) *Living with a seriously ill child.* Sheldon Press, London.

Claye, G. (2006) *Don't' let them tell you how to grieve.* WritersPrintShop. [Gina Claye is a bereaved mother. Her poems explore the emotions experienced by those who grieve.]

Dyregrov, A. (2008) *Grief in children: a handbook for adults,* 2nd revised edn. Jessica Kingsley, London.

Dyregrov, A. (2008) *Grief in young children: a handbook for adults,* 1st edition. Jessica Kingsley, London.

Gerner, M.H. (1990) *For bereaved grandparents.* Centering Corporation, Omaha, NE (www.centering.org)

Jenkins, C. and Merry, J. (2005) *Relative grief: parents and children, sisters and brothers, husbands, wives and partners, grandparents and grandchildren talk about their experience of death and grieving.* Jessica Kingsley, London.

Kissane, D.W. and Bloch, S. (2002) *Family focused grief therapy: a model of family-centred care during palliative care and bereavement (facing death).* Open University Press, Buckingham.

Klass, D. (1999) *The spiritual lives of bereaved parents,* 1st edn. Routledge, London.

Napthali, S. (2008) *Buddhism for mothers with lingering questions.* Orion, London.

Nouwen, H.J.M. (1997) *Bread for the journey: a daybook of wisdom and faith.* HarperCollins, New York.

Reed, M.L. (1999) *Grandparents cry twice: help for bereaved grandparents.* Baywood Publishing Company Inc., Amityville, NY.

Rosen, M. (2004) *Michael Rosen's sad book.* Walker Books, London.

Schwiebert, P. (2003) *A grandparent's sorrow,* 2nd edn. Grief Watch, Portland, OR (www.griefwatch.com).

Thomas, P. (2001) *I miss you: a first look at death.* Barron's Educational Series, Hauppauge, NY.

Index